ADVANCE PRAISE FOR *TURNING INWARD*

"*Turning Inward* is a wonderful invitation to engage more profoundly with our inner self, and it's a path to developing a meditation practice that can lead to contentment, creativity, joy, and a higher consciousness. It is a reminder that being in conversation with oneself can be a gift in these chaotic times."

—Lynn Nottage, Pulitzer Prize–winning playwright

"Witnessing his evolution from young yoga teacher to compelling spiritual guide, I know firsthand Ross's commitment to making these valuable teachings accessible. This book is a blend of intuitive wisdom, bravery, and sincerity. The only direction is inward, and Ross is the perfect person to light the way for us."

—Elena Brower, bestselling author and host of the
Practice You podcast

"Whether it's a morning yoga flow or an evening meditation, Ross's teachings ground me and help me honor the mind/body connection."

—Wilson Cruz, award-winning actor, producer, and activist

"*Turning Inward* provides the tools to befriend yourself. In sharing his mindfulness T.I.P.s, Ross provides a path for even the most novice meditator. Herein lie many entry points back to oneself."

—Robin Arzón, *New York Times* bestselling author

"I have worked in the wellness world for over thirty years, and what I love so much about Ross's approach is that he lives, eats, and breathes what he talks about in *Turning Inward*. His primary objective is to help people, to guide people with so much positivity and just to put good into the world. And he does that here, helping you to open yourself to slowing down and turning inward."

—Bob Harper, *New York Times* bestselling author

TURNING INWARD

The Practice of Introversion *for a* Calm, Joyful, Authentic Life

ROSS RAYBURN

with EVE ADAMSON

hachette
BOOKS

NEW YORK

Hachette Go, an imprint of Hachette Books
Hachette Book Group
1290 Avenue of the Americas
New York, NY 10104
HachetteGo.com
Facebook.com/HachetteGo
Instagram.com/HachetteGo

First Edition: January 2024

Published by Hachette Go, an imprint of Hachette Book Group, Inc.
The Hachette Go name and logo is a trademark of the Hachette Book Group.

The Hachette Speakers Bureau provides a wide range of authors for speaking events. To find out more, go to hachettespeakersbureau.com or email HachetteSpeakers@hbgusa.com.

Hachette Go books may be purchased in bulk for business, educational, or promotional use. For information, please contact your local bookseller or Hachette Book Group Special Markets Department at: special.markets@hbgusa.com.

The publisher is not responsible for websites (or their content) that are not owned by the publisher.

Print book interior design by Bart Dawson

Library of Congress Control Number: 2023948309

ISBNs: 9780306832444 (hardcover); 9780306832444 (ebook)

Printed in the United States of America

LSC-C

Printing 1, 2023

To Sally Kempton, for guiding me into my heart.

CONTENTS

YOU'LL BE OKAY

Many years ago, before I got interested in yoga and meditation, I was pursuing an acting career in Los Angeles. I was at a stage in my life when I didn't have much money, and even though I was starting to have some success, for the first time in my life, I was experiencing the anxiety of an identity crisis. I didn't know who I was. Was I on the right path? Did I have any value?

I had felt stress in my life before that, but there was something about that time in my mid-twenties, when I was starting to feel the pressure of success and living up to the expectations I had set for myself before I turned thirty, that caused my stress to escalate from youthful ambition to something more existential.

The worst moments were when I almost booked a part in a TV show or movie that would "change my life." Just so you know, in TV and film, getting an audition with producers is one of the last stages before you get the part. So whenever I got a producer audition, even though I couldn't really afford it, I would pay my acting coach, Shawn Nelson, for a private session.

One time, I was going in front of producers for an Aaron Spelling show, which was a big deal back in the 90s. I called Shawn. Sitting in his living room, at the end of one of the run-throughs, he looked at me in a way that I'd never seen before. It was a fatherly look, like he was going to say something important. He said, "You know, you're going to be okay."

At first I laughed it off. But then he said, "No, I want you to really hear what I'm saying. You realize, if you don't get this job, if you lose your agent—in fact if you never get any acting job again—you'll be okay." It was a mike-drop moment. I don't think I fully understood it at the time, but I did recognize that he was saying something profound.

It was the first time in my life that I was struck by the idea that my happiness was not dependent on my success.

Of course, it was about more than happiness. It was about my self-worth, contentment, and even my capacity to love and be loved. I think it became such a pivotal moment in my life because he managed to pack so much wisdom into the simple phrase: "You'll be okay."

The other reason why this was such a powerful moment for me was that growing up, I *didn't* think I was going to be okay. When I was young, I often didn't feel like I belonged. In fact, I often felt unwelcome.

I grew up in a loving but typical Texas Southern Baptist family in the 1980s. We went to church a lot and, to be clear, I loved going to church. I loved the fellowship, the community, the music, and I loved the celebration of God. But I felt alone and I was often told that

I would be alone. The people saying it didn't know that they were talking about me, but they were.

Even though I hadn't accepted it yet, I knew I was gay. At the time, I didn't even understand what that word meant. I simply felt "other" or separate. It took years of studying many religions, philosophy, and eventually immersing myself in the teachings and traditions of yoga and meditation, to realize that I wasn't separate. I was just different.

I think this was one of the main reasons why I started to pull away from the church. I loved so much about it, but I knew that at least temporarily, I was going to have to go somewhere else to find joy and fellowship.

I do want to say clearly that this was just my experience with my church at that time. There are a lot of churches that make a point of including the LGBTQ+ community, but there are still a lot of churches that don't, and I hope that will continue to change.

When I went to Southern Methodist University in Dallas, even though my degrees were in political science and journalism, I took a bunch of courses on religion and philosophy. I had always been drawn to philosophical thought, but my primary motivation was to understand why the god that I loved didn't love me.

Thanks to a couple of brilliant professors, I began to see that He did. I was still in the midst of a very painful coming-out process. Most nights, I kneeled by my bed and prayed that God would change me. But the seeds of being okay had been planted.

My first big job out of college was as a flight attendant on an airline that flew to South Africa, based in Washington, D.C. I took the job because I wanted to live in New York and try my hand at becoming an actor. I loved the theater, and had done some in high school and college. Even though D.C. wasn't New York, it was closer than Texas. Working for the airline and having some distance from home helped tremendously in being able to live authentically.

After the airline shuttered, and a brief, miserable stint in New York as an executive assistant, I moved to Los Angeles to give the west coast a shot.

Los Angeles was many things, but one of the best things was that it was a conducive and supportive place to come out in the mid-90s (the great fortune of meeting my first boyfriend, Alfredo, and joining his wonderful family of friends was also a huge help). I'll never forget sitting in a bar with a hundred other people watching Ellen De-Generes come out accidentally over a loudspeaker.

Then, in 1997, Alfredo and I decided to do an AIDS Ride, a charity fundraising bike ride from San Francisco to Los Angeles. I raised over $10,000 and from all the training, felt physically stronger than I'd ever been in my life. Unfortunately, I didn't listen to my body when my knee started hurting, and somewhere along the ride, I tore the meniscus in my left knee.

After a few weeks of being on crutches, letting it heal on its own, my friend Felix Montano said to me, "You should do yoga to rehabilitate your knee." At the time I thought yoga was only for women and people who were bendy. Little did I know it would become one of the great loves of my life.

I started taking yoga as often as I could. I studied with pretty much every teacher in the Los Angeles area. In late 1998, after I told my friend Howard Sussman (without him asking) how to improve his Warrior 2 (a yoga pose), he sweetly and snarkily said, "Maybe you should be a yoga teacher." So I signed up for a teacher training at

Yoga Works with Maty Ezraty and Lisa Wolford. Frankly, it was way too soon for me to be teaching yoga. I should have gotten a lot more experience first, but I was still in a hurry.

Then, a few years later, I took a workshop with John Friend, who had just started Anusara Yoga. John had a magical way of weaving spiritual ideas into the physical practice that I loved, and it reminded me of the spirituality I had so treasured in church in my youth.

John's use of a spiritual theme throughout a yoga class made practicing yoga less about preparing the body to sit for meditation—which is a common understanding of yoga—and more about celebrating who we are and practicing how to be better. It completely changed the way I experienced yoga.

A fire had been lit. His way of teaching, his theme-weaving, felt like the first time I pierced the barrier between the physical and the spiritual. I think like a lot of people, I constructed all sorts of barriers in my life. I mostly understood who I was by how I was different. John's way of breaking down the wall between the physical and the spiritual started me on the path of being able to break down my own barriers. It felt like opening a curtain on a window, revealing a world full of hope.

For the next few years, I dove headfirst into studying with John and a few other Anusara senior teachers like Desiree Rumbaugh. John was a touring yoga teacher, so in order to study with him, I had to go to wherever he was around the world. For the next three years, I went to one of John's workshops about twice a month. I put myself into debt, trusting and hoping that what I was learning was a career investment.

At a workshop in the fall of 2000, surrounded by three hundred fellow yogis, I remember John teaching about the importance of clawing the floor in downward-facing dog so that your wrists have more power and lift. This instruction was very personal because I had a lot of wrist pain at the beginning of my yoga practice. But he didn't just say, "Press your finger pads down and claw the floor." He said, "Press your finger pads down and claw the floor, as a way to honor your teachers. Do you want to do it lightly, or do you want to do it passionately?" I've always been passionate about gratitude, particularly towards people that have helped me, and so it blew my mind how much stronger I clawed the floor when it was about honoring someone rather than healing my wrist. Even thinking about it now makes me get emotional. It may sound hyperbolic, but it was life-changing.

John also taught meditation during his classes and workshops, and to be perfectly candid, I hated that part. I thought I was so bad at it. I even thought that I couldn't do it—that it was beyond my capacity. But I did it anyway, and even started teaching it, because that's what a yoga teacher is supposed to do. I was teaching meditation "by the numbers," using other people's words—it was a practice from the outside in, rather than something that flowed from the inside out.

Then, through John, I was introduced to Gurumayi Chidvilasananda (who you might not know you've heard of—she was the guru that Elizabeth Gilbert went to India to study with, in her book *Eat Pray Love*) and through Gurumayi, I met Sally Kempton. Sally, after a renowned journalism career in the 1970s, moved to India and became Swami Durgananda, then returned to the West, again using her given name, to teach meditation. Sally became my primary meditation teacher.

Meeting Sally was fortuitous for so many reasons, but foremost she showed me for the first time that it was possible to enjoy meditation. So much of why I didn't like meditation was that sitting still was difficult for me. I've always had a lot of energy and being still was terribly uncomfortable. I would get easily agitated. She taught me that it's okay to be comfortable—that even though good posture matters, it's okay to use props, pillows, and the wall for support. When your back starts to hurt or your foot falls asleep, it's okay to stretch. Her invitation to soften my perfectionist instincts opened the door.

That's when my own practice really took off. When meditation stopped being something that I had to do, when it became less of an obligation, I started to enjoy it. And I started to experience the many benefits of meditation I'd always heard about.

It was about this time that teaching yoga and meditation became my full-time career. I owned a studio for a while in Los Angeles, and in 2007, I too became a touring teacher, travelling around the world. Primarily, it was because of the global growth of Anusara Yoga that I was able to teach internationally. Over the years, I started to focus my workshops on biomechanics and therapeutics, helping yoga teachers know what to say when someone came into their class with an injury or some pain. And at the same time, my meditation practice was deepening. My therapeutic workshops increasingly included elements of my meditation, and I saw in my students how impactful meditation, attitude, and intention were in the healing process.

Then, in September of 2018, my phone rang. It was Kristin McGee, a well-known yoga teacher who had taken one of my workshops years before. She called to ask if I might possibly be interested in getting off the road and joining the team at Peloton, which was about to launch yoga and meditation on the platform. What I didn't say at the time was that not only was I interested but the constant travel was beginning to wear on me. By the time I started at Peloton, I calculated I had flown 3.3 million miles in twelve years. So I said yes.

With Peloton, my whole world changed. I remembered how wonderful it was to stay at home. Chris Wheeldon (my husband) and I were able to get a puppy. I got to go out to dinner with my friends on a weekend night. However, teaching on the Peloton platform felt a little bit like learning how to teach all over again. For twenty years, I had looked to the students in the room to guide me on what to teach. What did they need? How could I help them? But at Peloton, I was teaching to a camera. Sure, I knew there were students on the other side of the screen, but it was a whole new ball game.

My greatest fear teaching virtually was whether I'd be able to teach meditation authentically without the guidance I depended on by sensing the energy of the people in the room. Serendipitously, my meditation teacher, Sally, happened to be in New York around that time. She came over for lunch and I told her about my concern. She said, "Well, let's do one of your meditations." Of course, the thought of this terrified me. Have you ever recoiled at the sound of your own voice on a recording? Well, imagine what it felt like to not only hear my own voice, but see myself teaching meditation, while meditating with my teacher! But I did it, knowing it was a huge gift.

At the end of the meditation, Sally turned to me and, with her characteristic sublime simplicity, she said, "Just meditate. If you drop in and connect, spirit will do the rest." She was affirming that what I found inside would be received by the people meditating with me in the best way possible. That gift not only gave me the freedom to teach from my heart on a virtual platform, but I believe it was also the gateway that gave me the freedom to write this book.

I've spent years thinking about self-improvement and the dizzying number of ways we as humans can get in our own way. We're great at getting stuck. Getting unstuck—at least I can say this for myself—takes practice and skill. I've also spent a lot of time thinking about the inner self versus the outer self—what we see when we look in, and what we project to the world. One of the great revelations of my life was realizing that when the inner and the outer selves are more integrated, we can go from being stuck to being free.

I'm sure you can think of many times when you felt in the flow. Things just clicked. You could do no wrong. That kind of flow state is where we wish we could all be all the time, but the reality is, we all get off track, we all get stuck. That's life. Turning inward is a way to find some freedom and a tool for doing life better.

My hope is that you come to recognize that turning inward— what I call introversion—is not something foreign. You don't have to wait for years, like I did, to get it. This book is about all the ways you can crystallize, amplify, and get better at entering the flow in your own life. Even when the external world doesn't fit or stops functioning or doesn't happen the way you want it to, inner peace exists for all of us. And sure, there will be times when someone helps you, but you can also get there on your own.

I hope by learning to turn inward, you too can find something within you that helps you to know, like Shawn taught me in that audition private session, "You'll be okay," even if nobody ever tells you.

Ultimately, the path of introversion is about connecting your inner you with your outer you, connecting you with everyone else, and in fact, seeing connection in all things.

What you will find within is a salve, and sometimes a remedy, for self-doubt and insecurity, for separation and regret, for anxiety and stress. Through the practice of introversion, you can learn to recognize yourself and be that person more often, no matter what the world demands. This is a path to being all that you can be... which is to say, all that you already are.

CHAPTER 1

LET'S TURN INWARD

Turning inward—what is that? Is it contemplation, self-reflection, or simply thinking about what you're going to say before you say it? Is it preferring your own company or wanting alone time? Is it traditional meditation? Or is it all of the above?

Also: turning inward towards what, and for what purpose? You might think of yourself as a natural extrovert and enjoy spending most of your time focusing on the outside world and other people. You may genuinely enjoy your private time now and then, but you may be "allergic" to turning inward, happy not to look behind the proverbial curtain of your own thoughts, not to mention anything like meditation. You might even think you couldn't possibly meditate. You're too energetic. Your thoughts are too busy. You don't like sitting still!

But guess what? No matter who you are, how you think of yourself—introvert, extrovert, shy, outgoing, quiet, loud, calm, energetic—even if you've had no experience with any kind of structured contemplation or meditation, I am here to tell you that you already turn inward. In fact, I would even go so far as to say that at least according to my definition, you already meditate.

Everyone does it, consciously or not, in one way or another. You may not realize you're doing it, but whenever you unplug, de-stress, zone out, or do something to escape, you're responding to an instinct to take a break from your routine, to switch direction, or to relieve the uncomfortable feeling of stress. You're turning inward because you have a natural impulse to balance what you do most of the time, which is to engage with the external world. Out of necessity, you send your attention outward, and out of necessity, sometimes, you go the other way, turning your attention inward.

Maybe you have a glass of wine at the end of a stressful day, to feel more relaxed. You might do some yoga to feel more grounded or do something creative like write or draw. It could be binge-watching your favorite show, or scrolling through your social media for an hour, just to think about something else. Or maybe you just lock yourself in the bathroom and cry. Every single one of these things is a form of turning inward.

I often refer to myself as a yoga and meditation teacher, but all I'm really teaching people to do when I teach meditation is how to look within. To me, that's all meditation is. I also call this the practice of introversion (which I'll define in more depth later in the chapter), but for now, I want to share the simple and exciting idea that turning inward, in all its forms, is more natural, simpler, and more accessible than you may have ever realized.

I love people's reactions (particularly people who think they can't meditate) when I tell them that they are actually already meditating. One time when I was interviewing my fellow Peloton instructor Becs Gentry for a program she had created, she asked me how she could learn to meditate. She said that every time she's ever tried, she hasn't been able to do it.

Becs happens to be a top-level marathoner, and I asked her if, when she runs, she has ever gone into a flow state. She said absolutely. I had her describe it to me. She said she goes to another place. Time stops, or feels effortless. She describes the feeling as powerful and peaceful.

That's when I told her, "Guess what? You're already meditating."

I was shocked to see how excited she got because she never thought of herself as a meditator, even though she was well aware of what a flow state feels like when she runs—that feeling of a time-lessness, an enhanced ability or a state of ease, a state of mind that's seemingly above doubts and fears.

Becs's impression of meditation is like most people's. Almost everyone assumes that to be able to meditate, they will have to sit still and stop their thoughts. That's just not true. A flow state is a flow state, no matter how you get there, and we all have access to the deep and largely unexplored inner terrain familiar to regular meditators.

Think about times when you've experienced a flow state, or a feeling of unity, or sensed a higher consciousness, or had a moment of intuition, or experienced any state of mind when confusion turned to clarity. Maybe you were writing, or making art, or doing yoga, or having a deep conversation with someone, or going running, like Becs does. For most people though, these alternate states of mind seem to happen randomly. They often surprise us when they arise. Most of us can't just switch on a flow state, or enter a flow state on purpose. But it is possible, and turning inward is one of the best ways I know to access that effortless, timeless feeling of clarity and insight.

Learning how to turn inward purposefully is powerful. While in some moments it may seem like the least natural thing to do—like in an argument, or when someone bumps you in a crowd, or when you're stressed and exhausted from a long day—it's not difficult to learn how to take a moment to pause and look within, whenever you feel overwhelmed by life, or are feeling reactive or angry, anxious or frustrated.

Turning inward isn't always about profound moments. It can also be practical. It's a way to mitigate stress and find a way to handle a situation better, from a perspective of more lucidity and wisdom. Looking inside yourself taps into your knowledge and experience, so instead of reacting in a difficult situation, you can choose a more effective response. Knowing how to do this gives you a great advantage in human relations and the management of your own emotions. It's almost like having the high ground in a battle. ("Anakin! I have the high ground!" Any *Star Wars* fans?)

In fact, this practice can be the gateway for you to experience not just better interactions and less stress, but even revelations and joys. The place you access when you turn inward contains an infinite source of wisdom and calm for navigating life, and it's yours to access.

As I've said, turning inward is also the way I describe a practice I call introversion. Most of us think of ourselves as introverts or extroverts, but I use these terms a bit differently. In this book, introvert and extrovert are not character traits. They aren't something you are, but something you do. I use introvert and extrovert as verbs, not nouns, and both modes, both actions, are available to us all, no matter what our personalities are.

Introversion is simply the practice of shifting the direction of your attention from focusing on what's going on outside of yourself, to focusing on what's going on inside. It's like turning the proverbial camera around. Most of our day, the "camera" of our attention is facing outward. Most of the day, we look outward out of necessity. We extrovert (the verb) but turning inward points the lens within. It reverses, even just for a moment, the outward direction most of us send our attention, most of the time. And that can feel like a great relief, when the outside world becomes exhausting, stressful, or just too much input.

So you already introvert, but you can learn to do it more intentionally, for much greater benefits. Introversion accesses the inner you, and I believe the inner you contains all the wisdom you could ever need in life. Who you are inside is valuable and likely under-utilized. Your inner landscape can be a great source of insight and inspiration. There is a whole world inside of you that is vaster than you may realize—more comforting, more supportive, and more fulfilling than the external world often feels. For that reason alone, introversion is a skill worth cultivating.

INTROVERSION FOR GREATER AUTHENTICITY

Introversion can help you know yourself better. Without regular access to that essential you, you may not feel like you really know who you are, or what you're here for, or what you should be doing. If you've ever felt frustrated, anxious, angry, or adrift, without precisely knowing why, or if you ever have moments in your life when you just don't know whether you are doing the right thing, or you question your purpose, take heart. Living authentically is one of the great challenges of being human, but the search for authenticity is also supremely human.

The problem is that when our focus is largely external, it can be difficult to get a good sense of who we are. We all probably think of words like "authenticity," "integrity," and "being yourself" as good things, but when we think about what it means to really be authentic, we find it's trickier to figure out how to do that or what that means. We can't just flip on an authenticity or integrity switch—at least not when we aren't sure what those qualities would be. Authenticity doesn't come easily in our extroverted world. In fact, many people will openly admit, when pressed, that they feel inauthentic much of the time.

Feeling inauthentic can take many different forms. It can happen when you doubt yourself, or when someone criticizes you or says something negative. It can happen in a moment when you wonder if you're in the right job, or relationship, or whether you've made the right choices in life. It can come in the form of a nagging inner voice that says the person you are presenting to the world is not who you really are, or who you think you should be (or who you've been told you are).

Most of us know some versions of these unsettling feelings of inauthenticity. We often mask moments of inauthenticity with anger, sadness, and fear. We may feel anxiety, confusion, or depression. But what feels really, invariably good is when we discover a bit more of who we are, which can make authenticity feel more accessible. It can give us resolve, direction, even contentment.

Introversion provides clearer understanding of the many projected selves and our constructed outer presentations, as well as our more fulsome inner self. This perspective is a gateway of authenticity. You can begin to see that projected selves aren't false. Not only are the parts of you all you, but there is an inner you that is the sum of all the parts. Knowing *that* version of yourself better adds dimension, subtlety, wisdom, and yes, authenticity, to all the parts of you that you project to the world.

So how do you do this? How do you begin to discover a bit more of who you are? How do you know when you're being genuine, and when you aren't? Turning inward is the best strategy I've found. I'm still discovering ways to turn inward—it's a practice for a lifetime—but turning inward has truly changed my life, and I think it can change yours, too.

FROM MEDITATION TO INTROVERSION TO TURNING INWARD

I've already suggested that turning inward is a kind of meditation, so to be clear about that, I'll tell you an origin story.

For much of my life, I struggled with the idea of meditation. As I mentioned in the introduction, as a yoga teacher, I felt like I should have a meditation practice, and I sometimes led guided meditations in my yoga classes, but sitting and meditating was extremely difficult for me. I didn't like sitting still, I had trouble focusing, and I definitely couldn't stop my thoughts. I thought meditation was some mystical doorway that was supposed to transport me from one reality to another. Sometimes I experienced a bit of calm or an altered state of some kind, but it was random and fleeting. Most of the time, I just didn't get it.

Then, years ago in a lecture, one of my teachers, Carlos Pomeda, used the term "introversion" in place of the word "meditation." He was explaining the many different forms meditation can take, and he made the point that meditation was really just looking within—his definition of introversion.

I remember this clearly. It was a light bulb moment for me. The idea of meditation as introversion felt more inclusive. It felt accessible rather than intimidating, and to me, it made more sense. Just replacing that one word, meditation, with a different word, introversion, began to change the way I thought about this practice. In my teaching, and also within my own mind, I started using the word "meditation" less, and the word "introversion" more. And the concept seemed to resonate with a lot of my students who struggled with meditation.

Fast forward to discussions with my publisher about the title for this book. Originally, I wanted to call this book *Thinning the Veil*. This is a metaphor I like to use because I often imagine that what divides us from others and from ourselves is like a veil that can be thick or thin, depending on our perceptions and experiences. Sometimes, the veil gets thicker, for protection or when we are angry or feeling less self-aware. Sometimes, the veil gets thinner when we have moments of clarity. Although it's a metaphor that doesn't always apply to everything I wanted to write about in this book, I liked the poetic sound of it.

When my editor suggested the title *Turning Inward* as an alternative, I was initially reluctant, admittedly attached to my working title. But the more I thought about it, the more I realized that not only was *Turning Inward* a good title—simpler, more direct—but it also achieves in a greater measure something that Carlos's use of introversion had done for me: it made meditation more accessible. It cast a wider net than any of the words I'd been using before.

Casting that net wider, for me, is one of the highest acts of service I have to offer. I hear all the time how the idea of meditation is intimidating or sounds too difficult. But the benefits of looking within are so large that I have made it my mission to make this more accessible and to help people see how easy it can be, and as I've mentioned, how most of us are already doing it, even if we don't realize it, even if we aren't doing it on purpose. I believe that inclusion and accessibility are crucial for establishing a consistent introversion practice. If it feels too hard or too complex or out of reach, people are less likely to keep it up, or even to try it at all. If they do try it, they may give up if the definition is so strict that it feels unreachable.

So even though turning inward is an unorthodox way of defining meditation, for me, it's worth bending the definition because of the doors it opens. The instinct I have to broaden the scope and make introversion more accessible is largely based on my own experience, and the frequency with which people tell me they are afraid to try meditation, because they don't think they can do it. *Sit on the floor. Keep your back straight. Close your eyes. Don't move. Don't think about anything.* That's not so easy. What if you aren't able to sit on the floor? (You don't have to.) What if you can't keep your back straight? (That's okay.) What if you can't keep your eyes closed, or stop moving? (Also fine.) What if you can't stop thinking? (I would argue that it's impossible to stop thinking.) What if your foot falls asleep? (It's okay to stretch your legs out.)

Thinking you're doing it wrong is the quickest path to quitting, which is why I want to emphasize to you right now that *you cannot meditate incorrectly.* Or, to make it sound even more approachable: *you can't turn inward incorrectly.* That's not to say it's always effortless, nor is it to say that different kinds of introversions have different benefits. They certainly do. But it's not something to be graded. It's just something you can choose to do—something that I believe can change your life. Understanding that it's easier than you think helps people feel like they can do it. This gives you a foothold to do it a little more regularly, and the benefits then get better and better.

I do want to make a point of honoring traditional methods of meditation. I have the utmost respect for people who practice within one of the ancient lineages or distinct meditation schools. If you are someone who leans toward a more traditional definition of meditation, as you read my liberal interpretation, I would ask your forbearance. Ultimately, my hope is that learning how to recognize moments of turning inward and how to turn inward more purposefully will make the whole concept seem a little less mystical, a little less "other," and will result in people bringing meditation into their lives.

THE EXTROVERTED WORLD

I've already talked about introversion as turning inward, but I'd like to further clarify it by exploring its opposite. Let's talk now about extroversion, or what it means to extrovert.

In this book, I use extroversion as a way to describe all the moments when we put our attention on something or someone outside of ourselves. In today's world, we're required to extrovert a lot. Whether you're looking both ways before you cross the street, chatting with the cashier in line at the store, posting on social media, or talking to your colleagues at work, you are extroverting.

Because of the myriad ways we must engage with and navigate the world, most of us spend the majority of our day extroverting. We listen to podcasts, we watch TV, we go out to restaurants or the movie theater. We walk, we drive, we talk, we laugh, we eat, we work, we interact. And this can be good and necessary. Extroversion allows for fun, safety, and relationships. What would we do without it? The very nature of living in communities requires extroversion, and extroversion is how we've created a culture of identities, activity, and narratives. All our stories are extroversions. We are creatures of story. We love to tell stories, we love to hear stories, and we often define who we are by the stories we tell. All day long, our attention is typically directed outward, telling our stories for the world to see and hear. We do specific things in order to show people who we are. We groom ourselves in a certain way, we wear certain clothes, we say certain words.

Think of all the extroverting we do with our devices and during our daily interactions. We constantly place our attention on our computers and smartphones, obligations and pleasures, colleagues and friends. And it's often transactional: the person at the checkout counter or the person driving the bus or the one bumping into you in a crowd requires an extroverted exchange of some kind. In each case, though, whenever we place our attention on something outside of ourselves, extroversion is inherently performative. That's not to say it's false, just that there is a practiced or improvised performance we exhibit in all those situations. This is important, but more on this later.

There's also an overlap where turning inward can become extroverted. We can even extrovert in our own minds—this is a bit more complex, but I do define extroversion to include not just outward attention but also inward attention that gets stuck on something that happened externally, or that could happen externally. Extroverting in the mind is directing your attention, sometimes obsessively, towards something you did, are doing, will do, or might do in the external world. For example, obsessing about a mistake we made or getting stuck in worrying about something in the future are forms of extroverting.

INTROVERSION BALANCES EXTROVERSION

To state it clearly: extroverting is necessary, and important, but when it crowds out all or most introversion, we can begin to forget that the self we project to the world is not the whole self. When the extroverted world gets to be too much, introversion is a way to relieve the stress, to improve the interaction, or just to take a break.

Being aware of which one you're doing and knowing how to shift your attention from one direction to another is a powerful facet of shaping the balance between introversion and extroversion (more on that later). But for now, think about how being myopically stuck in your extroversion, you could miss the solutions to your problems. Instead, what if you were able to pause and shift your perspective; that's when you're more likely to "see the field," identify patterns, and choose a better path. Introversion is like rising above the labyrinth of life in order to see the way out. As I've said, it gives you the advantage of the high ground.

One of my favorite words is perspicacity, which is the capacity to perceive patterns and to make connections that others might miss. Think about the people in your life that you consider successful, or think of great leaders throughout history. One of the things they likely share is a high degree of perspicacity. They may be deeply involved in the extroverted world, but they usually have a superior level of clarity and understanding, an internal insight underlying external action.

Perspicacity is something that you can cultivate and amplify in your life. You can be the person in the meeting that is able to rise above the seemingly unsolvable situation and offer a way out. You can be the person in your family during the holidays that sees a path of unity when everyone else seems stuck in irreconcilable division.

You can be the person who remains calm and clear-headed when everybody else is panicking.

Another big introversion benefit is that it taps into something we all possess: an inner source of wisdom and creativity. Think of a moment when you had an insight or a revelation simply because you took the time to ask yourself what to do. That's turning inward. I have an unwavering belief in your built-in wisdom. Of course, some people are more in touch with it than others, and of course, it can be cloaked and seemingly out of reach.

Philosophers and scientists have debated the source of wisdom for thousands of years. But I think of inherent wisdom like the sun. It is powerful and transcendent. In the same way that you don't doubt the sun's existence on a cloudy day, you shouldn't doubt your inner wisdom when it's illusive or dimmed. For that matter, I believe you can learn to trust your vast inner creativity, even if you may sometimes lose sight of it or can't seem to find it. It's in there. You just have to turn inward to find it.

These two benefits—perspicacity and creativity—are good in and of themselves. But there is something additionally great about increasing both in your life. When turning inward becomes a habit, especially when you start integrating a higher perspective and your inner wisdom into your life, a natural rejuvenation occurs. There's an affirmative momentum—you feel calmer, clearer, better, and more like yourself. You can achieve a deep feeling of authenticity and contentment.

I'm inviting you to turn inside and discover your own potentiality, in whatever way feels comfortable, natural, and right to you. I'll be giving you a lot of methods and options, but all you have to do is pick one and give it a try. Whether it looks like "regular" meditation or not, what matters is that you're turning inward, in a way that works for you.

And guess what? I don't want you to take my word for it. Your experience is the ultimate judge, not me. When it starts working, you won't need me to tell you. You'll know it's happening for you in the same way you know when music is harmonic or dissonant, or when you are moved by a piece of art, like a painting or a sculpture.

If you're unsure if you can find it, that's okay, too. I'm not worried in the least. One of my great beliefs is that your awareness of your inner self—its power and wisdom—is your destiny. Like the way water always finds a path through all barriers in its journey towards the ocean, the vast universe within will find its way through the barriers we erect. It might be in a dream or a flash of insight or a moment of catharsis or a burst of creativity. But whatever your gateway, I have faith that you will discover your true power.

INTROVERSION FOR HOMEOSTASIS

Introversion feels good after a lot of extroversion in the same way that sleep feels good when you've been awake all day. Introversion balances extroversion just as sleep balances waking. On some level, it's mysterious why balance is so valuable, but it probably has something to do with the physics and biology of homeostasis. Our bodies naturally maintain balance in all organ systems to keep us alive, and that may translate into benefits for all types of balance: physical, mental, even spiritual. To some degree, this is the mystery, and this isn't a book about homeostasis, but it's something to think about when you're feeling the need for more balance.

T.I.P.S: TURNING-IN PRACTICES

In this book, you'll learn a whole range of "Turning-In Practices," or what I call T.I.P.s. Some of them will be short practices you can do throughout the day. These are called Quick T.I.P.s. The regular T.I.P.s will be longer, more like traditional contemplations and meditations. I'll provide these along the way so you can begin practicing turning in throughout every chapter. By the time you get to the four-week program for building an introversion practice, you'll already know what you're doing. I highly encourage taking the time to try the T.I.P.s and the Quick T.I.P.s because habit building does help.

A note about the practices in this book: These practices are structured as guided introversions. These are always challenging to put into book form because I can't actually say them to you (unless of course you are listening to the audio version of this book). There are a couple of ways you can solve this problem. You could record these and listen to them, following along to your own voice. However, I get that not everybody likes to listen to their own recorded voice. In that case, I suggest that when you do these guided exercises, you read the first item, close your eyes, take some time to turn inward and consider it, then when you are ready, open your eyes and read the next bullet. Take as long as you want between each part. You may want to spend some time contemplating some parts of these practices for a longer time than others. It's your practice. Once you've gone through one of these introversions a few times, you will likely be able to do it without reading the prompts. This is an easy way to learn how to move in and out of an introverted state, and will work for every introversion practice or guided meditation in this book.

If you would like to keep a record of your introversion practices, you might want to start a journal where you can write about your experiences and how they made you feel. I suggest doing this especially if you like to write.

Here's your first Quick T.I.P. to try.

QUICK T.I.P.

This brief exercise is a way to think about any problems you are having, decisions you have to make, or issues you are trying to resolve. You may already know the answer. Turning inward can help you find it, or at least think about the issue from a different perspective. Before you do this exercise, make sure you are somewhere that it's safe to close your eyes for a few moments.

- Sit or lie down comfortably. Close your eyes. Take a few slow breaths.
- Think of a problem that you're dealing with, a question you have, or a decision you're trying to make. In your mind, put the question into one sentence, such as, "What should I do about…" Just ask the question in your mind. Don't try to answer it.
- Now, imagine that you are sunbathing on a beach. Let the question fade away. Feel the sand beneath you, the sun above, warming your face. Listen to the sound of the water or the wind. Picture yourself feeling calm and relaxed as you absorb the sun. Stay here for a few moments or minutes.
- Now, return to your question. Does the question feel different? Do you have a feeling that you know the

answer now, or are you leaning in a direction? You
might not have an exact answer, but notice if there's
a shift in how you feel about the question, as well as
how you feel in general. Are you calmer, less anxious,
clearer? Has the importance of the question changed
in your mind?

- If you want to start keeping track of your introversions,
write down your experience.

Now let's try a T.I.P. that's a bit more involved. This is an example
of the exercises you'll find at the end of each chapter. Don't feel like you
have to do these in any particular way. You can sit or lie down, stand
or walk while contemplating these exercises. If you feel uncomfortable,
you can move. You can take as long as you like between bullets—two
seconds, two minutes, or more. As with the Quick T.I.P.s, you can
record yourself reading these bullets, or you can read each bullet, close
your eyes, contemplate that step, then when you're ready, open your
eyes and read the next bullet.

T.I.P.:
INTROVERSION-EXTROVERSION EXERCISE

The purpose of this exercise is to help you get used to feeling the difference between extroverting and introverting, and to experience what it feels like to shift your attention one way and then the other. Know as you try this exercise that it is very natural and within our human capacity to both extrovert and introvert. Neither is good, neither is bad. All we are doing is bringing awareness around what each one feels like.

- Find a comfortable posture in a place where you can relax quietly for a few minutes.
- Close your eyes and take a few deep breaths. Slow down each exhalation, almost like you are rationing your breath. Spend longer exhaling than inhaling. Breathe this way for about a minute or so.
- Begin by extroverting. With your eyes closed, imagine the room that you're in, the door where you came in, the color of the walls, the different pieces of furniture that might be around you.
- Give some of the things you notice a label: say what they are, quietly to yourself. "Door, chair, rug, window."
- Now, switch to introverting. Imagine the space within your own body. Try to visualize the space inside your torso, and more specifically, the space where your internal organs are, like your heart.
- See if you can feel your insides, in any way at all. Can you feel your heart beating? Your pulse? Your stomach rumbling? Even if you can't actually feel your insides, try to imagine what they feel like.

- Now, switch back to extroverting. Think about the people you've seen today. Imagine you are in the moment where you saw them, and place your attention on them, as if they are there in front of you. Think about how they looked, what they were doing, where you were when you saw them. If you interacted, think about what you said and what the other person said.
- Now, switch back to introverting. Think about how you felt inside when you saw or interacted with people. Try to feel that inner feeling again. Ponder why you felt the way you did. Do you have an inner sense of the reason for your reaction to different people? How do you feel right now, remembering those people?
- Take a deep breath in, then a full exhale. Allow all the visuals to fade.
- Gently open your eyes.

CHAPTER 2

THE SEPARATION PARADOX

There are so many ways that we separate the world. We see each other separately because of course we are all individuals. Every person who has ever lived has been unique. We have individual bodies with singular experiences and paths. Humans also separate ourselves into groups. We are born into families; we place ourselves into communities. We've done this for centuries, for safety and to thrive as a species. And, as we already discussed, there is a separation inside each of us—a separateness between our different identities, between our deeper selves and our more projected selves.

At the same time, we are all connected. We're all human. We share this planet. And all of us have pasts and futures, hopes and dreams. There is also a strong argument that on a deep level, we are interconnected. There is a kind of unity. Ultimately, we are all one.

Granted, this is a spiritual or philosophical argument, but it's an idea shared by many (and one I personally believe).

So which is it? Are we all different, or the same? The answer is both. That's the paradox. I'd go so far as to say that calling it a paradox isn't even controversial. The true rub is reconciling the paradox. How do we hold these two opposite ideas in our heads at the same time? How do we simultaneously see ourselves as unified and distinct?

To be candid, reconciling this paradox is probably impossible to ever achieve fully, but we can get glimpses of it. Even the quickest of glimpses can be powerful. The more important point though is that these flashes of awareness are accessible to everyone, and with practice, we can learn to string together these glimpses so that they shift from being fleeting to being a sustained experience.

Reconciling the paradox, whether it's momentary or sustained, is one of the single greatest secrets in life. For me, it has been game-changing. I would go so far as to say that I wouldn't have achieved any of the success that I have without having been exposed to this concept.

Seeing division isn't hard for us, but seeing connection, and then seeing both at the same time, is unusual. That's why introversion holds so much potential. There is something about looking into the nebulous inner landscape that increases the aperture to see things as unified rather than divided. For instance, if you are in an argument with someone, a moment of turning inward can help you to see your common ground. Holding both the shared perspective and your own perspective simultaneously gives you the power to solve problems without surrendering your principles.

But again, it's easier said than done. Not only is it a challenge to perceive separation and unity simultaneously, but there is a similar challenge, even once we bridge the paradox, to then turn around and consistently integrate that multifaceted perception into the real world, where it has utility and adds to the value of our lives.

But it is possible! The practice of introversion will teach you how to see through many lenses, inside and outside, to perceive the ways we're connected and how to integrate all of it in your day-to-day, in order to thrive and live your life to the fullest.

There is a story I have very loosely adapted from the *Mahabharata*,* about three brothers who set out on a journey. The journey was long and strenuous. They were desperately thirsty when they came upon a lake. As they knelt to drink, a water goddess rose up and said to them, "Before you drink, you must answer a riddle. If you don't answer correctly, the water will take life, rather than give it."

The first brother stepped up. The goddess leaned down and whispered in his ear, "Who is here but not there, and there but not here?"

He searched his mind, but he couldn't come up with an answer. Overcome with thirst, he scooped up some water and immediately collapsed with the first sip.

The next brother approached. She whispered her riddle again: "Who is here but not there, and there but not here?"

The second brother searched his mind, then said, "I am here and not there, and you are there and not here." He knelt down to the water, drank, and immediately died.

The third brother stepped up and said, "Great goddess of the lake, I have a condition of my own. If I answer your riddle correctly, I will offer you a riddle, and if *you* cannot answer, will you bring my brothers back to life?"

---

* An ancient epic poem in Sanskrit that includes the *Bhagavad Gita*.

Sure that a mere mortal could not outwit her, the goddess agreed. For the third time, she whispered: "Who is here but not there, and there but not here?"

The brother searched his heart and said, "The worldly man is here but not there, and the spiritual man is there but not here." The goddess bowed respectfully. He then asked her: "Who among us is both here and there?"

The goddess, in her surprise, admitted, "I don't know the answer."

The third brother said: "The worldly man is here. The spiritual man is there. But the enlightened man is both here and there."

With those words, his brothers came back to life, and they all continued on their journey.

The moral of this story is that there is merit to being "here" in this world, and there is merit to being "there" in the spiritual world, but too much of either is not the ideal. The ideal is to be able to move between worlds with ease and intention. The worldly person over-extroverts. The spiritual person over-introverts. The more enlightened person knows how to do both, as needed, on purpose.

There are many examples of people who easily get fascinated and obsessed with success in the material world, and there are examples of people who get overly fascinated and obsessed with the spiritual world. But we can be both here and there. Sure, it's paradoxical, but I believe it's a paradox we can surmount.

The separation paradox can exist on many different levels—the separation of individuality, the separation between spirituality and materiality, and the separation between who we are inside and who we present to the world. In truth, this life is full of both separation and unity, the tangible and the ineffable, the known and the unknown. This practice is a way to give ourselves permission to think about these concepts in different ways and come at them from different angles in order to identify more fully with two important ideas: that (1) you are more than you might know, and (2) there is common ground for all of us, no matter how different we might feel or think we are.

Let's look first at how this applies to you.

THE TWO SELVES

Every one of us has a self, deep within. It is who we are at our core, it is our true nature, and it has always been there and will always be there. But each of us also has a self we project to the world. It may be a more careful, reserved self, or a louder, more confident self. It may be a version of us that feels it has to look a certain way or meet certain expectations. It is the self that everyone else sees and interacts with. The projected you is always somewhat different from the self that is deep within, simply because it's impossible to fully express our total truth in any given moment. In fact, the many facets to the outer and inner self can become so profoundly separated that we lose sight of their connectedness.

Imagine that you live on an island in the middle of the ocean. You only know the island and you've never been to the shore to see where you are. When you only know the island, you can begin to think that the island is all that exists. You can forget—or maybe you never knew—that you are on an island in the middle of a vast ocean.

Your daily consciousness is the self that knows only the island—it is how you think and live and act in the world. Most likely, your daily consciousness consists mainly of extroversions. But to introvert is like stepping to the shore and seeing the vast ocean—to realize that life on the island is not all there is. The ocean represents the deeper self—it is the source of your untapped creativity, insights, wisdom, even the indescribable and unknowable mysteries of consciousness. Introversion thus becomes a path from the island to the ocean.

However, most of the time, life is busy and you have to stay on the island getting your work done and living your life. You may not have a lot of time to stand on the beach and contemplate the vast ocean. We often default to what's necessary, or what's known and familiar. For instance, when we introduce ourselves to other people, we usually lead with one particular story or one particular version of ourselves. In a busy life, that can feel like the easiest way to get by. But it can be all too easy to forget that our limited, convenient, socially acceptable projected self is only one small part of who we really are.

The truth is, you have many identities and facets to who you are, and you likely have parts of you that you have yet to discover. Deep down, we know this to be true. Unfortunately, because of life, it's easy to get stuck in a limited view of ourselves. I'm guilty of this all the time, and it makes total sense why this happens to all of us. Just like routines and habits can become fixtures in our lives, the small, limited versions of ourselves can mask our ability to receive who we really are. When we're stuck in a small version of who we are, it can be painful.

One of the ways to recognize that pain is to think about it as dissonance. When you listen to music, you can recognize dissonance versus harmony, and when we are stuck in a smaller version of ourselves, but something tells us that's not who we are, we know that we're not living harmonically. We are living in a kind of dissonance.

This dissonance or fragmentation feels like being a fraud. It's the source of imposter syndrome—feeling like you're secretly unqualified for your job or undeserving of your success. It can be a source of anxiety, depression, or identity crisis. It can make you feel unsure about who you really are. It's exhausting and it can lead to feelings of overwhelm, burnout, emptiness, anger, fear. It can also be the withering away of joy and creativity as we get older.

To reiterate something from earlier: it's important not to vilify any of your identities or to be too hard on yourself if you feel stuck in just one of your stories. Remember that extroversion is important, necessary, and rewarding in many ways. The different parts of you are still you. The trick is to remember that these parts are not the full you. It's imperative that you remember there is always more—in fact, there is more depth within than you may ever fully uncover.

Stepping onto the path of remembering and discovering, seeing your different identities as connected, and looking within to explore and uncover more of who you are, is a joyful journey that can yield a multiplicity of benefits like contentment, compassion, and creativity.

Imagine a prism. When you shine a light through a prism, the prism splits the light into individual colors. Those colors are like the projected versions of you. But, the rainbow side of the prism is all coming from one light source.

When you think about yourself, are you thinking about just one or two versions of yourself, like only seeing one or two colors exiting the prism? Or do you see your whole self, both in the full spectrum of the rainbow, and the light source entering the prism? Being able to see all of it as you is essentially bridging the gap between who you are inside and the many selves you instinctively or judiciously present to the world.

We have the capacity to remember that there are always other colors or facets of ourselves that exist beyond the one that we might be presenting to the world, and we can remember that the individual colors are part of a more holistic inner self. The reason this matters is that remembering lessens the chance that we might get stuck in one particular identity or one narrow narrative.

The reality is that because we all get into routines—we're predominantly presenting one or two, maybe three or four parts of our personality each day—it makes sense that we would forget about the less often presented parts of who we are, not to mention forget about the source of where those identities all come from.

I'm a good example of this. I slip into a limited view of myself all the time. I teach on the Peloton platform, where I am literally projected onto my student's screens. And while I try to be open, honest, and real about the many different versions of who I am, it's still a curated version of me. So when I turn inward, I try to look for patterns in my life that are becoming ruts. I look inside and try to detect ways that I'm stuck—things that I might not have noticed without introversion. By turning inside, I'll sometimes detect something that might not be a big deal. For instance, I might notice I've started teaching the same lesson too frequently or I've been using one version of me as an illustration too often. By recognizing this early on, I'm decreasing the chance that it turns into a deleterious, limiting pattern. Instead, I can make a shift and grow.

Another possibility is that when we present ourselves to the world at any given moment, we might not be choosing which facet of ourselves to present, but we are most likely choosing a default version that we know seems to work in that type of situation.

This can be useful. Can you imagine if we presented our whole selves every time we met anyone? Imagine having to listen to your work colleagues spill all their personal secrets. Imagine having to listen to everything about someone on a first date—their whole life story, all their opinions, all their preferences, all their hang-ups. What would be left to explore and learn? Would you *ever* go on a second date?

In society, we've even constructed general rules around greeting each other. Typically, when you meet someone in a casual or inconsequential setting, and you ask, or they ask, "How are you?" we usually don't take that as a serious probing question on our true state of mind. We usually hear that as a polite way to greet each other. We are expected to filter our answers according to the situation in a socially appropriate way. If we meet someone we know, or someone who is for some reason interested in more than a superficial greeting, then we may answer the question with more detail. If it's someone we don't know well, we're probably going to default to the socially appropriate answer, out of courtesy.

With introversion, even if it's a quick look inside to open to other facets of who you are, you can suddenly bring into that real moment and add to that default version other layers that create depth, complexity, and sometimes even sensitivity because the quick turn-in has a way of slowing the momentum of the default self. In other words, you end up presenting yourself with a little bit more presence. People often pick up on that sensitivity. That can deepen your understanding of yourself and others, and it can deepen other peoples' understanding of you.

QUICK T.I.P.

Take a moment right now to stop and think about all the versions of you. Can you name some of the many versions of yourself? Make a list of all the "yous" and spend a minute or

two feeling your incredible multiplicity. See if you can visualize
that behind all of those parts of you, which are all legitimately
different in character, there is a deep inner you that encom-
passes all the versions of you that you've ever projected. Sit
quietly, eyes closed, softly breathing, and see if you can get
a feeling, even just a glimpse, of that wise inner light that I
promise you have within you, and how it gently fuels every
other version of you.

THE SELF AND THE OTHER

If all introversion did was help you to be more authentic, more fully
you, it would be well worth your time. But there's so much more.
Another profound benefit to introversion is how it can help us connect to each other and find more harmony in an often divided and
unharmonious world. In the same way that our inner and outer selves
often feel separated, our identities and our individuality naturally
make us feel separate from each other. But this doesn't have to be a
problem. It's important to recognize how identity and individuality
are built into every facet of life.

We identify in distinct ways—genders, ethnicities, jobs, age
groups, pretty much any way we describe ourselves. *I'm a lawyer.*
I'm an artist. I'm a teacher. She's smart. He's funny. They're sexy. Self-
identity is primary. Learning more about who we are is one of the
most natural urges we have as humans. That's why it feels so good
when you learn something about yourself that feels true—when you
embrace an identity that's authentic. Don't we all love a personality
quiz that helps us identify more about who we are as individuals?

Also, when we tell stories, we use individual characters. We couldn't tell a story without separating one character from another. We use protagonists and antagonists, villains and heroes, jesters and tricksters. In a good story, not only are there distinct characters, but they're usually clearly defined. In other words, they're not just separate. They're unique. In fact, when we're telling stories, we lean into separateness to achieve that uniquity and clarity.

And don't we love stories? What would we do without them? Stories have great power to teach us things. They can reveal things that might resonate with us and solidify how we see ourselves. And in fact, stories have the power to reveal profound inner truths that can be guideposts in our journey of self-discovery.

Similar to how stories and myths have the power to teach us deeper truths through the use of characters, our individuality is necessary in daily life. One of the other primary human needs beyond self-knowledge—arguably more primal—is survival. And while in today's world survival means something very different depending on your socioeconomic status, everyone has probably had an experience of danger, where their survival instinct kicked in. If this has happened to you, you have felt how primal this is.

I don't have kids (although I have two puppies), but I bet if you have kids, you absolutely don't need me to explain the survival protection instinct. It would be ridiculous to propose seeing the interconnectedness of all humans in a moment of extreme danger. The survival instinct will kick in, and you do what you need to do. This is both right and good. Of course, there are heroic examples where individuals thought of others beyond themselves first, but it's important for us to recognize that there's nothing wrong with our built-in, deeply innate self-interest to survive.

A more light-hearted example of this is competition. I love to compete and have been accused of being a bit too competitive at times. If somebody says "game night," my hand is the first one up. I also love sports, and anyone who loves sports understands the joy that competition can yield. We certainly wouldn't want our favorite tennis player or our favorite race car driver to be connected rather than to be competitive. But when does competitiveness or survival stop being affirmative and slip into harm or get in our way because it's too egoistic?

I realized my own competitiveness was a problem when my husband, Chris, would never want to play games with me. I tended to take all the fun out of it because I love to win. It was a problem. What I've learned to do—a way of introverting to solve this problem—is soften my edge a bit when we play games. And, I've learned how to not be so disappointed if we do something other than game night. I'm sure you can think of ways you could shine more self-awareness on your tendencies in your relationships.

To be clear, I'm not a professional in any kind of relationship field, but I am a huge believer in the importance of having quality relationships in life.

We humans long for connection. It's an essential part of our innate desire to thrive and make our lives meaningful. We long for someone to understand us emotionally, to touch us physically, and to engage with us intellectually. We need to feel supported and lifted up.

You might be in the camp that argues "opposites attract," or maybe you believe that we look for partners and friends who share characteristics of our identities. If we were all the same, none of that would be possible. This goes for any relationship you can imagine—friendship, life partner, family.

We first have to see ourselves as separate in order to discover connection, in order to build relationship, and in order to recognize similarity and possibly even unity. It only becomes a problem— and arguably our biggest problem—when we are so stuck in our identities that we lose the will, the strength, or the agency to get beyond them.

QUICK T.I.P.

Next time you have a conversation with someone, pause without them knowing, and say to yourself some phrase that's true about something you share. It could be, *We're both standing in this store together. We're both wearing blue. We're both made up of bones and muscles.* Anything that establishes connection. Have a brief moment of recognition before you engage in conversation, and then once the conversation is done, make a mental note of your experience.

When we're stuck, we're only feeding our mind's wondrous capacity to separate things and forgetting to feed our capacity to see how things are connected. Getting stuck turns into lost or lonely. This is where the power of turning in reveals its magic. Just like our ability to look inside and remember more of who we are before we present a part of ourselves, we can also look within and remember how we're all connected before we interact in the many ways we do throughout our day. And it truly seems magical how different a conversation can go when there's a moment of introversion and subtle recognition of connection before we engage with someone.

TRIBALISM AND POLITICS

The last mode of separation that I'd like to highlight is the way we separate ourselves into groups. Stop and take a quick inventory of all your different groups. There are community groups, family groups, religious and spiritual groups. There are groups that share interests, like teams, regions, and nations.

Working for Peloton, one of my favorite things has been to see all the different organic groups that exist—#physicianmoms, #black-girlmagic, #broadwayfans, #boocrew, #powerzonepack. A group of my students call themselves #fullblastfam (I say "full blast" a lot, and FULL is an acronym for ferocity, unity, light, and love).

We use a lot of words to connote group connection: families (even when it's not people we're related to), communities, teams. In today's politics, we often refer to groups as tribes. An important aside: This word is problematic because it can appropriate ancient and traditional tribes. However, I use it here because it's a fairly well-understood term. My intention is not to offend.

The simple reality is that it feels good to be supported by a group of like-minded souls. In fact, community has many benefits. It's rooted in an ancient need for security, which an insular, supportive group of people provides. It's why society formed tribes and civilizations in the first place. Groups build confidence and can confirm our views about what's right and wrong.

One of my favorite phrases is, "You're preaching to the choir." I certainly do it all the time, and my hunch is that in our siloed world, that's true for most of us. Preaching to the choir can be coded negatively, but it also can have value. The benefit of preaching to the choir is that it's a way to get consensus or build momentum around an idea. You're talking to your "base." This can be a unifying, even strategic tactic in business, when you need to build consensus, particularly when you're asking people to make a change.

If you're working with a group of people whom you're about to ask to go with you in a new direction, especially when that new direction is potentially arduous, it would be unwise to demand change quickly or immediately. However, if you invite them into a recollection of shared values and goals, you reinvigorate their spirit with how much you all share. Also, you're articulating how much you all have already accomplished. This establishes a much stronger foundation from which you can then ask them to join hands and take a leap of faith in a new direction.

A couple of things are accomplished. First, you acknowledge and honor those who have been around and who have done the work. And, you create unity by directing people's attention toward shared experience. Just like there is power in remembering the unified self, there is power in reminding people of their inner-connectedness. It's that power that drives our capacity to change. For good or for bad, we are all built for herd mentality. Or, to state this more elegantly, unified consciousness.

The negative version of preaching to the choir (or even just the benign version) might be a little bit more obvious. You've probably said, "Quit preaching to the choir," to someone because it seemed unnecessary, inflammatory, or simply indulgent. It's a natural impulse we all have to be validated and have our beliefs reflected, but the potential of it becoming an echo chamber—siloed off from other perspectives—has negative consequences. This has always been the case when it comes to politics, but it seems like we're in a particularly acute period of preaching to the choir. Whether it's the internet, twenty-four-hour news, or globalism, it seems like the characteristics of our time have conspired to make this an inordinately turbulent moment.

For me, it's concerning but not apocalyptic. To be sure, I am keenly aware and don't want to minimize how much fear and anxiety people experience when politics comes up.

From the time I was a little kid, I loved politics. I fondly remember my family dinners when politics would come up. That continued through high school and college. One of my college degrees was in political science. At the time, I wanted to become an attorney and maybe eventually go into politics. Of course, life had different plans for me, but my passion for politics hasn't faded.

When I first started studying meditation, I would have never thought there would be a relationship between the subtle realms of the inner self and the pugilistic world of politics. But not only is there a relationship between them, politics in its highest form is a product of inner awareness.

The main reason my love for politics is even deeper than it was as a kid is because what I've learned by turning inward has helped me to remember that politics is ultimately about service and community. I don't want to be cavalier about the anxiety we have around politics. Seeing unity in the face of difference, or remembering service and community when there is need and suffering, should not be oversimplified. Depending upon your level of privilege, your relationship to politics can range from casual interest to life-or-death. And I think that's why people are so passionate about their beliefs. I respect that. However, that doesn't solve the frustration when we are entrenched in our camps, often feeling powerless, without agency to make a difference or a change in the world.

I firmly believe that one of the most potent ways to make change is to access our capacity to look past the thickest walls of separation and remember what we share, so that we start from a place of community before advocating for change. It can sometimes seem impossible to find connection, let alone unity, with groups of people we don't understand or even openly detest. Our default is usually to simply find fault and assume malicious intent wherever there is disagreement.

To be clear, I am not advocating for dimming or diminishing your voice or your passion. I'm not asking you to soften your beliefs. I would never suggest anyone abdicate their right to fight the good fight. But when we first recognize what we share, we can enter those fights with greater awareness and a keener sense of fairness. Moreover, our beliefs are more likely to create change when we first tap into our capacity to remember what we share. Our voice becomes less abrasive and more persuasive with the presumption of connection.

Admittedly, this is massively easier said than done. I've practiced this for years and I still find myself piqued, even angry, in the face of disagreement and injustice. But that's when we have to remember that turning inward is not a panacea or a universal solution to every problem. It's an opportunity in even the most fraught moments to find something within that could provide more agency and efficacy in the real world.

Beyond politics, beyond relationships, even beyond the complex journey of self-discovery, the separation paradox is about recognizing both the one and the many as both unified and distinct. It's easy to forget the context in which we all exist, when immersed in the simple act of living our lives.

ARE YOU A SKEPTIC?

Skepticism is a tool. Without it, we would be completely gullible and vulnerable to manipulation. Skepticism is like an alarm bell alerting us to be mindful about whether something we are hearing or saying or buying into is right and true. A healthy skepticism can alert you that you are introverting too much and losing sight of what's going on around you. It can alert you that you are fixating on something external and forgetting to check in with yourself. An unhealthy skepticism can turn into cynicism, where you suspect everything and lose all trust and faith in your own intuitive sense of what's true.

I've been through periods in my life when I didn't have a healthy skepticism—I didn't always want to turn over the apple cart or rock the boat so I just went along. If you're having a good time on the boat, why would you want to rock it? It feels good to preach to the choir, to be accepted, to have things be familiar. On the other side, you can go too far into skepticism to the point where it crosses into cynicism. If you're black-clouding, even when things are going well because you're making great choices, your skepticism might stop the momentum that you've built up.

Skepticism is putting checks and balances into your own day, process, and perception. Generally, skepticism is introverting—I just want to be sure you can also be skeptical of your introversion. It's an introversion on an introversion. It might be recognizing that you're introverting too much and you need to get out and play. Essentially, as a seeker or as a person who's interested in navigating life, a healthy skepticism is a barometer for what you're doing in your life and what you believe. Use it to keep you grounded, but don't let it bury you.

CAN WE SOLVE THE PARADOX?

The short answer is no. Not to be glib, but if there was a solution for it, it wouldn't be a paradox. I do believe that we have the capacity to navigate the paradox better or more skillfully. We can cultivate our ability to hold the many disparate and apparently separate parts of life and consciousness in an ever increasingly sophisticated way. I would in fact argue that experience, wisdom, and often just age are sources of doing what I like to refer to as "bridging the paradox."

The bridge metaphor is imperfect, as are all approximations of esoteric concepts, but it does fit for many of the different ways in which introversion turns our attention toward a perspective with a keener vision, in which we can become more able to perceive the "landscape" and thus more able to navigate or cross the paradoxical divide.

You could say that when we create or perceive a bridge between things that are seemingly disconnected, that's when we can experience a shift in terms of emotional state or even in a sense of agency and empowerment. Since we are usually extroverting or seeing things as separate, introverting is a directional shift, and it's the shift that creates the bridge. This is a tricky concept. Chapter 3 explores this more fully.

Sometimes the shift inward is to balance out all the extroverting we do, and sometimes it's more about stepping into our ability to widen our view and open to inner wisdom. We'll cover examples of how and when and where we bridge the paradox more passively or instinctually, and also with more intention and precision.

But here's one of the most important ideas in this practice: the more you recognize the separation paradox and how introversion and extroversion can be bridged so that we can consciously cross back and forth, the more familiar it will become. And the more familiar it becomes, the more comfort you'll experience. Along with comfort comes ownership and, potentially (if you choose), mastery. And that's when you can not only change the trajectory of your life, but become a beacon of light and hope for everyone you meet.

In the next two chapters, we'll dissect the why and how of turning inward to explore our inner "neighborhood," and we'll move down the path towards familiarity and mastery. In order to get to know our bridges and the way introversion shows up in our lives, in chapter 3, we'll dive a little deeper into the reasons why we might introvert. In chapter 4, we'll go over some of the specific ways we can introvert more often and with more awareness.

To close this chapter, I'd love to share with you one of my favorite parables about the separation paradox. Two young fish were swimming along together. An older fish swims by and says, "How's the water?" The two young fish respond quizzically, "Water? What's water?"

Most of our day is spent swimming, sometimes with, sometimes against the proverbial current. But one of the greatest gifts of introversion is the expansive perspective to recognize the current, the swimming, and our shared ocean. The young fish and the older fish actually represent endpoints on a spectrum, from pure extroversion to full awareness. Outside the fable and in the real world, we exist in multiple places of awareness on that spectrum, depending on the innumerable variables of life.

T.I.P.

A really simple way to think about introversion in the face of complex relationships with groups or even concepts is encapsulated in the axiom "Think before you speak." If you feel the urge to react, take a beat, turn inward, and look at the situation through the lens of your internal knowing. What do you feel? What might the other person feel? What is the response most likely to move you forward? At first you might think you don't know the answers to these questions, but even a moment of introverting, during which you ask yourself, *What words will help?* can help you to possibly respond very differently than if you hadn't taken that beat. And what an example you will be setting. Just imagine a world where all of our projections were supported by introversions. Surely we could understand each other better, we might be more compassionate to each other, and we might spend less time on things that don't matter—and more time on things that do.

CHAPTER 3

BRIDGING THE SEPARATION

If I had to pick one way to describe why we need introversion, it's because we humans tend to get stuck. We get stuck in patterns, we get stuck in our learned view, we get stuck in restrictions that are either built in or systematic or just somehow are the result of where we ended up in life. The reason we don't want to remain stuck is because every single one of us wants to grow and be free. As I've mentioned many times, introversion isn't a cure-all, but it can be useful in either helping us get unstuck, or at least mitigating the suffering, whether it's simply discomfort or something more serious or even traumatic.

In the last chapter, I mentioned that introversion builds bridges in two ways: (1) by shifting our familiar tendency of extroverting or focusing our attention outward, and (2) by placing our attention on the inner landscape, to gain a different perspective. But first we need to ask: How do we know we're stuck? Let's start there.

Sometimes, our stuckness isn't evident, even to us, unless we turn inward and recognize a feeling of being off. Often, if we really go inside and feel it, it's a feeling of being dissonant.

Essentially, dissonance is a ripple of asynchrony that can cause a feeling of dysregulation and difficulty. You can feel it in the body, and you can experience it in your thought process, in the same way you recognize whether music is off-key. Sometimes that dissonance feels like a vibration or a motor running in the body. In the mind, dissonance can feel like excessive mental chatter, worry, obsessive thoughts, hyperactivity, perseverating, catastrophizing, or fear.

It can also feel like sadness, pessimism, apathy, inertia, lethargy, anger, irritation, or simple mental discomfort, like the feeling that something bad is going to happen, even if you can't quite place what it is. It can feel like a loss of confidence, an identity crisis, or hopelessness. You could see anxiety as a sped-up asynchrony and depression as a slowed-down asynchrony. Either way, your rhythm is off, and you can feel it.

Whatever the mental dissonance, you already have an antenna for it. No matter what your mind is doing, some part of you knows whether it feels right or wrong. It's not so much what you're doing, but how it feels for you. You can hold multiple opinions in your mind at one time, and that might not feel dissonant to you. You can hold on to a single opinion and it can feel dissonant to you. The litmus test is the feeling of asynchrony.

Some people are in a state of asynchrony all the time, with chronic feelings of panic, burnout, overwhelm, confusion, grief, low self-esteem, lack of confidence, overconfidence, arrogance, or excessive ego. With a regular introversion, you can build a bridge between dissonance and synchrony, just by going inside and searching for what feels off.

Anything you do that has an inherent rhythm to it can bring resonance. Maybe it's running as fast as you can, or walking at a steady pace. Maybe it's going dancing. You could get quiet and listen to some music, or just sit and feel your own breath moving in and out. Just know that somewhere inside of you, even if it feels very deep and far away, there is a space that is quiet, and you can go in there if you choose. At its most primordial, just find the rhythm of the breath. Once you have recognized dissonance, you can begin to find ways to bridge the separation that caused it.

FIND VALUE FIRST

One of my influential yoga teachers, John Friend, came from a system of yoga that was passed down to him in which a common tendency of the teacher was to point out what students were doing wrong, in order to teach them. He created Anusara Yoga partly to institute a system that pointed out the good first, and then the correction. He used the phrase: "See the good." In my own teaching, I changed that to "See the value" because I think "good" has so many potential interpretations and the word "value" is more precise in terms of its usefulness. What is valuable to one person may not be valuable to another, and value can apply to both successes and mistakes, joys and even tragedies.

I try to practice this principle in all aspects of my life, and I believe that after recognizing dissonance, the next step is to introvert to find the value in whatever you're experiencing. This is a powerful practice that can be almost like a superpower. Go inside to find the teachable moment, the value others don't see. When you're in a stressful situation, it can feel incredibly difficult to pull back and see the value. You might not see it right away, but learning to plumb the depths of your dissonance in order to find value is one of the highest forms of introversion.

The reality is, you can be good at introversion generally, but you also need an alarm bell to make you aware when you feel off, and that it is an opportunity to build a bridge to remedy the separation and find unity.

QUICK T.I.P.

If you're feeling off, pause for a moment and take a deep breath. Close your eyes if you are able and see if you can feel where in your body you are feeling the discomfort. Maybe it's physical pain, or maybe it's a tightness in your head, chest, or stomach that signals stress or anxiety. See if you can relax into the tight area and open it up. Breathe into it. Even if you aren't entirely sure where it's coming from, turning into it and breathing into it can help that dissonance to relax and release that part of your body to get back into synchronization with your normal pulsation.

BUILDING THE BRIDGE

Between any two sides of a separation, there exists the potential to build a bridge. Bridging the separation paradox maintains the separateness of two things (inner and outer self, self and others, groups and other groups), but finds a way to cross over, shift direction, or change perspective in order to find common ground.

Familiarizing and demystifying introversion as a bridge-builder can help you build momentum towards making introversion a habit, and increase the chances that you'll choose to introvert intentionally more often. This may feel a little awkward at first, to build a bridge from somewhere you know to somewhere you don't know, or don't know as well. I liken this to how it feels to do a new workout. It's always a little more difficult to do something you don't usually do because of the unfamiliarity, but as something becomes less foreign, a momentum of ease sets in.

Think about the first time you ever drove through your neighborhood when you first moved somewhere, and the feeling of unfamiliarity, the discomfort of not knowing where you are. Once you get to know your neighborhood, familiarity transforms your experience of the neighborhood, even though the neighborhood itself hasn't changed.

What does building a bridge by introverting look like when you actually do it? Sometimes turning inward to build a bridge feels like changing direction, shifting from an extroverted perspective to an introverted perspective, or even from an introverted perspective to an extroverted one. Sometimes building a bridge will feel more like a stepping back, a shifting of perspective. A wider view. You can build a bridge from where you are to where you would like to be. Anything that facilitates empowerment or agency is a bridge from less-than to more-than, a bridge from deficit to abundance.

Sometimes the shifting of direction and the wider view will inspire you to act, or shift your action. Or, it might confirm that you should continue with the same action, or make the same choices, but you'll be doing it more consciously and you'll be able to see

more clearly why you're doing what you're doing. Sometimes introversion is a bridge to what you would naturally do versus an alternative perspective or action. Sometimes the bridge is a bridge from
the superficial myopic instinctual reactive perspective and self, to a
slower-thinking, wiser, perspicacious ability to see patterns.

You can build a bridge to a higher perspective, or it can be a
two-way bridge traversing the internal and the external. Or it might
be more like the mechanism on a railroad that shifts the direction of
the track or diverts your momentum to a different track.

All these versions of bridges involve some level of introversion
because it is by turning inward that we can most easily find the
unity inherent in separation, and that is what we can use to build
the bridge. This is how introversion as a bridge helps us move from
natural separations, particularly when they are problematic, to connection. Introversion can be a remedy for the discomfort, the disad-
vantages, and even the suffering that can occur when we either view
or live from a limited or separated perspective. It can be a strategy
to get unstuck. It can alter the perspective or ease the discomfort or
change the dynamic of any situation.

THAT BEING SAID . . .

Turning in can often be a remedy for getting stuck in patterns, but you can turn in and get stuck as well—you can
get stuck inside of yourself, ruminating and filling with self-
doubt and frustration. That can lead to a downward spiral
of self-criticism. I would argue that there is still some value
in that—at least you are looking in and trying to find the
answers. But no one wants to cultivate self-doubt, and it

is possible to get lost in there if you don't come back out and remind yourself where you are and what you're doing. Instead, if you can keep thinking of introversion as a bridge rather than feeling like you're creating a black hole, that's when the benefits start to become clear.

Beyond the immediate and utilitarian benefits of bridging separations, there is often some calm and joy that arises as resonance sets in. But there are other specific benefits. Here are some of the practical ways bridging the separation paradox can be valuable to you.

INTROVERSION QUIETS THE NOISE

Building a bridge between our extroverted world and our introverted self can be a way to escape stressful situations, or at least the worry that surrounds them. Remember that glass of wine or scrolling or bingeing a TV show—those are introversions that are responses to the instinct to go on a mini vacation. They might not be the deepest or most ultimately fulfilling ways to introvert, but when you do them consciously, in healthy amounts, they can be effective introversions. Remember that since we spend most of our day extroverting, looking outward and not inward, there is something satiating and beneficial in our attention going in a different direction than it normally does. Sometimes, you can accomplish that by zoning out and shutting down to the outside world in whatever way is easiest for you in the moment. It's like crossing a bridge from a bustling city to a quiet retreat.

INTROVERSION SLOWS THE MOMENTUM

Building a bridge can feel like slowing the momentum of a situation when you feel like you're on a collision course or like you don't have control over your words or actions because of anger, frustration, or just going too fast. Introversion can slow you down and create a pause, making a space in which you can choose to change perspective, change direction, take a different approach, make a better choice, or just get more clear on what you're saying or doing. In this case, the bridge is directional—the bridge can help you change your trajectory, so instead of charging in one narrow direction, you can pause, stop, and possibly turn around and go the other way.

If you're in an argument, for example, without introverting, it's very hard to suddenly stop your mental trajectory and say "Okay, you're right and I'm wrong." You can't just turn on a dime. The extroversion of arguing has a velocity to it and in fact, you could argue that it's both good and natural in an argument to have momentum. Tug-of-war is about increasing momentum to win. I remember a tug-of-war at camp one time when someone suggested on the count of three, everybody briefly stop and then restart. This surprised the other team so much that they all fell over, then our team was able to pull and win. That little pause—a kind of introversion—changed the game.

Building a bridge with introversion can do the same thing in an argument—not necessarily as a trick to win, but as a way to pause and reflect on what you're saying and what the other person is saying. By stopping your momentum, you might see the value in an alternative point of view. You might be able to have a moment of reassessment about what you're arguing, how important it is, or why your approach isn't working. Slowing the moment shifts the perspective.

GO TO BED ANGRY

The first time I heard someone say that it's actually better to go to bed angry, I was both shocked and relieved. I had grown up with the opposite idea as true. The point of this surprising advice was that oftentimes when we're angry, we're so stuck in the feeling or the tangle of the argument that we can't see a way out of it. Sometimes, the best way to reset and ultimately find a way past anger is to just sleep it off. Sleep, like introversion, can be a reset. The bridge from waking to sleeping puts us into a new place, where we can see things from a different perspective. This is an instance when introversion and sleep share some territory. Turning inward will not necessarily solve all your problems—and neither will sleep, necessarily—but it can soften the grip your problems have on you, and that can make all the difference.

INTROVERSION HELPS YOU DETACH

When you're mired in the thick of a situation and you're attached to the outcome, it's harder to have a higher perspective, but building a bridge from attachment to detachment can help you rise above that thicket and feel less attached to your position or what's going to happen. Even if we don't consciously realize it as attachment, it's human nature to attach to things that we think or see or feel because we've made a connection to those things. Routines, habits, preferences, possessions, opinions, addictions, people—these are strong forces and sometimes the attachment to those things can feel unbreakable. However, when we build a bridge from attachment to detachment, we can rise above the intensity of the attachment and see it from a higher perspective. The bridge from attachment can lead to potential empowerment and agency, as we gain more self-awareness around the nature of our attachments. Building this bridge may not change your advocacy or direction, but at least you're gaining some insight into your advocacy or direction, from an elevated, more holistic perspective. The diminished boundary between what you think you must have and what you see that you don't necessarily need or can let go of might even help you to make a better choice than the one you were aiming towards—possibly a less self-interested, more generous choice.

TEMPORAL ATTACHMENT

Attachment isn't just to people and things. You can also become attached to time. When we are in a situation—when something is happening to us *right now*—it can feel like that thing is always going to be the way it is in the present moment. The suffering we feel, or the joy, the relationship or the possession, the experience or the hope for an experience, can all feel endless. We want, or we don't want, the experience to end and we think it won't. We fear our current suffering will last forever, or we dread that a joyful experience will end. One of the bridges you can build through introversion is one of temporal detachment. You can shift to a higher temporal perspective in order to realize that even though something may feel like it will last forever because it's happening now, there was a point when it didn't exist, and there will be a point at which it won't exist anymore. This can break the hold a situation has on us. It can give us hope. It can help us to let go. It can set us free from attachment.

The apparent feeling of permanence is nothing more than an attachment to the present moment. Building a bridge from the finite to the infinite can completely change how you are dealing with a situation. You can see that your suffering will not last forever. You can see that even though a joyful experience will end at some point, you can be filled with gratitude for the gift of that experience, and wonder at what might be coming next. You can essentially step out of time, or above time, to a boundless, formless place where you can gain perspective about the nature of your attachments.

Here's an example. I'm not sure whether it was something I was told or something I concluded on my own at some time in my youth, but I grew up thinking that I wasn't good with money. I became attached to the notion that finances and my relationship with money were always going to be a problem in my life. It wasn't until I began to turn inward more often and contemplate this strange idea I had that I began to open up to a different perspective on money. That changed my relationship with money as I began to detach from the notion that I wasn't good with it. I was then able to develop a more positive relationship with money. The fear I had around it, the way that I talked about it, and the financial choices I made began to change.

You can probably think of your own examples of some idea or habit you're attached to. There are innumerable examples of this. We all have very real attachments, actual physical attachments, and perceived attachments, in every aspect of our life. Of course, we won't be able to loosen every attachment through introverting. But if an attachment is problematic, introversion can be a way to regain agency over your relationship with that thing you are attached to. Particularly with attachments that are negative, like addictions that are harmful, introverting (on your own or through the help of a guide, a therapist, or a doctor) and viewing that attachment from the perspective of the interior landscape can be the beginning of a shift. It's easier said than done for sure, but well worth trying.

INTROVERSION TEACHES YOU THE ART OF CONTEMPLATION

How often do you make time to really sit and contemplate something? We're all so busy making sure our brains stay busy and stimulated that it seems increasingly rare that we just sit and think about things. Introversion can build a bridge from distraction to focus, where contemplation can take place. You can go to a space that is more likely to inform you or remind you that there is more that exists than whatever you're doing in the external world. There are other facets of who you are that you could choose to express. There are other things to know than what you already know. You can explore who you are, simply by opening up to the question: *Who am I?* You can explore what you know, simply by opening up to the question: *What do I know?*

It's harder to discover things about yourself when you're in the momentum of action and routine and conversation and pattern and old stories. You can certainly discover things about yourself through action and through conversation, but ultimately it's those little moments of reflection, or longer moments of contemplation about your actions and conversations, that are really the source of discovery and growth. Opening the aperture of reflection and contemplation helps you to view your reality as not just a result of your choices but as a treasure trove of potentiality. Trust that you can look inside and strike oil. Just as we trust that the earth has reservoirs of oil, we can look inside with that same kind of hope and belief that we can tap into reservoirs of beauty and wisdom and goodness, just by taking the time to do a little mining.

INTROVERSION OPENS YOU TO MYSTERY

Mystery in the movies is great. Mystery in our lives can be stressful. However, there is power in the unknown. Think about when you were a child and knew almost nothing. You were a blank slate, a sponge. Children learn other languages more easily. They soak up life and want to know and understand everything around them. It's why they ask so many questions. As we get older, the brain starts pruning and our knowledge gets more deeply entrenched. We have opinions and preconceived notions, stories about who we are and who others are. We have an idea of what our lives are, what reality is. When you look at things in the external world, your brain fills in the blanks of the unknown, like what we can kind of see in our peripheral vision. We fill in the information we don't have based on previous experience, rather than being open to new experience.

But there is beauty and joy in cultivating what is called the beginner's mind. You can access this state through introversion as you build a bridge between the known and the unknown. Inside, you can cross over into the unknown and open to what you don't yet know. The inner landscape, when cultivated, opens us up to the truth that we don't know everything. You could discover something absolutely new that you've never felt or experienced or chosen. That is one of the most powerful aspects of a childlike curiosity—to break out of old patterns in order to become open to potential, to other ways of seeing, and to other choices. With introversion you can go inside and step into an open, spongelike acceptance of the mystery you possess within. It can change the surface of your consciousness from hardened and stubborn to porous and dynamic. In a way, it's like a spiritual fountain of youth.

To get there, you can begin by first practicing the assumption of mystery. Remember that no one knows everything. There is always more, so stepping back from knowledge and what you've already learned, opening up to the mystery of what you don't know, sets the ground for insights and creativity, and the beautiful magical experience of inner revelation. And as esoteric as this might all sound, it's actually super useful in the external world, when you're faced with a problem, a moment of uncertainty, or a creative dry spell. In that open, unknown space, you can discover a voice of insight, creativity, and wisdom. It's your voice. You can then look within for answers that seem to come out of nowhere but are really coming from your own deeper self.

T.I.P.

There is a teaching that there are four winds that send our mind out of the present moment. They are nostalgia, regret, anxiety, and hope. Those are the four ways that we spend the majority of our mental time. This concept was life-changing for me. Learning this made me much more aware of when my mind is caught up in one of these non-present states, and this helped me to be present more often.

You may be wondering what's so bad about hope and nostalgia, even if you recognize that it's not always mentally productive to feel regret or anxiety. We do generally code hope and nostalgia as positive states of mind, but in terms of the four winds, they actually have a negative element in that they are not present. Then again, who says you always have to be present? You can argue for the positivity of all four of these states, rather than slip into the common tradition of meditation books to only value the present moment. Even regret and anxiety can have their place as they are signals from your body or mind that there is a problem to deal with.

I think it's great to practice mindfulness, but I don't think it is a "should" scenario where you put pressure on yourself to achieve the impossible state of 24/7 mindfulness. The human mind doesn't work that way. It scans through time and emotion for a reason, and even if you don't always know the reason, you can trust that there may be value in sometimes being out of the present.

Think about where your mind is right now. Are you feeling nostalgia? Regret? Anxiety? Or hope? And how often do you slip into these states? I learned to set up a little mental alarm bell that goes off to alert me: *Hey Ross, you're in regret mode.* This alone is a bridge to jumping back into the present. If you can begin to bring awareness around where your mind is throughout the day, you can access this bridge. To do so, introvert to find where your mind is and what it's thinking about.

INTROVERSION INCREASES PRESENCE OF MIND

There is incredible power in presence of mind. Many great books have been written about the power of being in the now. Sometimes this is called mindfulness (and I use that term, too), but I like to call it presence of mind because that alludes to the sense of being present in the moment. Sure, it instantly becomes the past, and the illusiveness can be frustrating, but the more you practice and sense being in the moment, the more you'll notice an increase in clarity, efficacy, and even power.

Being present can even feel like a superpower. Navigating change because you're not stuck in the past, honoring relationships by truly listening to people you're with, even solving problems because you take in more facets of a situation, are just some examples of the presence-of-mind superpower.

T.I.P.: CULTIVATING THE SKILL OF INTROVERSION

You can begin cultivating your introversion skills right now by building bridges between inner and outer, known and unknown, separation and connection. I've already given you various quick turn-ins and exercises at the end of the first two chapters, but the very first step to introverting is simply tuning in. You can turn in to tune in, just by noticing what's going on inside of you. Imagine you are a radio and you are tuning in to the station that most clearly broadcasts a signal from your interior landscape.

You can do this at any moment throughout the day, sitting or moving or talking or working. Glance inward every so often and tune that dial. What are you feeling physically, emotionally, mentally, or spiritually? Since you're probably already introverting throughout your day, not necessarily on purpose, get curious about when and where and why you're already doing it. Be alert to when you tend to do it naturally. Do you spend a few minutes in bed in the morning after waking up, thinking about how you feel, what's on your schedule, or setting an intention for the day? That's introverting. Do you take a lunch break and sit quietly contemplating while you eat, or take a walk outside? That's introverting. Your weekend hobby might be your introversion refuge.

As you begin to become more aware of when you naturally introvert, become more intentional around your introversions:

- Intentionally introvert more often in your normal day.
- Intentionally put some of the quick tips or other introversion practices in this book into your day, where they didn't exist before.
- Make note of how you feel when you introvert. Do you feel different than you did before you introverted? Does your day go differently when you introvert more often?
- Note at the end of the day or week, either literally writing it down or just making a mental note, about things that happened that might have gone better, or differently, had you introverted first.
- Talk about your introversion experiences and your practice with people who you think would be interested and receptive. Let people know what you're doing as a way of crystallizing your own practice.

CHAPTER 4

VEHICLES FOR INTROVERSION

Introversion can be as simple as pausing and taking a breath, but there are many ways to introvert that are built into our lives—in fact, built into our very bodies. Recognizing these spaces we inhabit as opportunities for introversion is a way to embrace them and increases the chance that you'll introvert more often because you are already doing the things that can take you inside. From the physical (like your own body) to the metaphysical, here are the vehicles for introversion that are almost certainly a part of your life.

YOUR FIVE SENSES

Perhaps the most natural vehicle for introversion is your senses. The senses work from the outside in. They are your body's way of interfacing with the world. You see, hear, smell, taste, or touch something in the external world, and your brain immediately interprets the sensation and often evokes a reaction based on what's going on internally. To use the five senses as vehicles for introversion only requires becoming conscious of how you react internally to external sensory impressions.

YOUR INNER LANDSCAPE

One of my favorite ways to think of the spaces or the innumerable places you can put your attention within, is to see them all as part of a vast inner landscape. Sometimes when you go in, your view will seem like a familiar reproduction of an outward view, like imagining yourself on a beach or creating an image of a fire to help focus and shift your perception. And sometimes, when you go in, it can be formless. This will depend on what works for you in any given moment. Sometimes when you turn in, the inner landscape will have definition and clarity, and sometimes it will be more like bathing in your own experience and awareness.

You might even come up with another term to describe the subtle realms of your inner self, but I encourage you to see it as a fertile, unlimited, and mysterious source, so that there is always the assumption that it holds more than you already consciously know or possess.

T.I.P.

To introvert through your senses, try this introversion that scans through each of the senses and moves from outside to inside. You can do this quickly, or take your time with it, depending on how much time you have and how long you want to spend exploring your five senses as a mode for introversion.

1. Sit or stand comfortably in a place where it's safe, and close your eyes. Take a few minutes to shift from the outside world to the inner world.

2. Take a few deep breaths to help focus your awareness, then imagine all your senses except your sight are temporarily turned off. Open your eyes and look around you.

3. Notice everything you see, not as known objects but as shapes, textures, colors, levels of brightness and darkness. Notice light and shadows, movement and stillness.

4. Turn inward and notice how you feel as you concentrate on your sense of sight. What kind of physical, emotional, or mental response are you experiencing?

5. Now, close your eyes and imagine all your senses except your hearing are temporarily turned off. Listen intently and intensely to everything you can hear. You don't have to tag it as a particular sound. Just let the sound flow into you.

6. Turn inward and notice how you feel as you activate your sense of hearing. What is your body's response? What is your mind's response? What feelings and sensations do the sounds you hear bring up for you?

7. Keeping your eyes closed, imagine all your senses except your sense of smell are turned off. Notice anything

you can smell, obvious or subtle. If there aren't any strong smells, it may take a moment to register as you really home in on your sense of smell. (This sense is typically less developed in people who can see and hear.)

8. Turn inward and notice how you feel as you encounter different scents. Do you have any response to them?

9. Still keeping your eyes closed, imagine all your senses except your sense of taste are turned off. Do any tastes linger, from a meal or snack, or a cup of coffee or tea you've had recently? Do you taste toothpaste? What does your saliva taste like? Really focus on what you can taste, even if it's just the taste of your own mouth.

10. Turn inward and notice how you feel as you encounter any strong or subtle taste sensations.

11. Finally, imagine all your senses except your sense of touch are turned off. Without reaching out to touch anything, feel everything you can feel that's touching your skin. Feel your clothes. Feel your shoes. Feel your hair. Feel the air on your skin, and anything else that is touching you—the floor, a chair, a bed, a wall.

12. Turn inward and notice how you feel as you encounter the sensations of physical touch. What comes up for you as you focus in on this sense?

13. Slowly open your eyes and see if you can get a sense of feeling all your five senses at once. Note that you do this every day, but usually not with such heightened awareness.

14. Note if you feel different than you did before this introversion.

15. Bonus introversion: See if you can carry a heightened sensory awareness throughout the rest of your day.

YOUR WHOLE BODY

It might sound strange or untrue, but we don't actually spend that much time inside our physical bodies—or at least, most of us don't. Except for times when you were in pain, when was the last time you really focused on your insides? If the last time was never, you're not alone. It might even be news to you that you have the capacity to think about this at all.

QUICK T.I.P.

Using your body as a way to introvert starts by simply pausing, taking a breath, and noticing how you feel inside. Don't worry if you aren't sure how much you're supposed to feel, or if you're feeling exactly the right or accurate thing. What you feel could be physical, like discomfort or ease, or mental, like worry or excitement, or emotional, like sadness or joy. Just start trying to feel it. Start in quiet moments—how about right now?—and direct your attention inside. If that feels new, that's okay. Just try it. You can't do it wrong. You'll begin to glean the benefits of introversion from this practice alone, even if you don't do anything else from this book.

Or, if doing this feels familiar, you can turn your attention inward to your physical body and start to ask a few simple questions: *Do I feel grounded? Does my physical body feel open? Do I feel present inside my body or does my body feel like something separate from me?* You can begin to ask yourself these questions now, either as your initiation to tuning in to your body, or as a way to buttress your already realized physical introversion practice.

Everybody is a little different in how they will respond to what they feel. When they are stiff, some people need to slow down to navigate the stiffness, and some people need to move more, to almost dance. The major point here is the question: Are you listening? For instance, are you noticing whether you are stiff or loose throughout the day? When you notice, you are empowered to respond from a conscious place, rather than reacting from an unconscious place.

INTEROCEPTION

Proprioception is the capacity to perceive the physical body in space, and interoception is the ability to perceive the inner space or internal world of the physical body. Proprioception is a kind of extroversion, as we relate to our environment, but refining interoception is the subtle ability to perceive what's going on inside, not just from the sensations that most people feel, like hot and cold, pain and pleasure, but the more subtle things we all feel, when our muscles are tight, our joints stiff, or when we have the freedom of an increased range of motion. Interoception is great for introverting to find the source of physical discomfort, but it can also signal when our bodies are responding to nonphysical internal forces like stress, worry, anxiety, or depression.

Think about the signals your body might be sending you: A prickle on the back of your neck when you think you might be in danger. A stomachache when you're about to present something to a group of people. A bad feeling when you walk into certain spaces. Even a tension when you are around someone who exudes a lot of negativity, or an ease when you're on a great date or deep in conversation with someone. Interoception can even be a great friend finder.

Whenever you recognize yourself in an interesting conversation with someone you don't know, go inside, imprint it, recognize it, and make a note of that person, to possibly invite them into your world or maybe invest in spending more time with them. Or, if your interoception is telling you to go another way, you may want to avoid that person in the future.

When you refine your interoception, you can become like a trained musician who hears every nuance in a symphonic performance, versus someone who simply hears the melody. There is a whole catalogue of benefits—physical, mental, even spiritual—to amplifying and elevating how skilled we are at listening to what's going on inside.

In fact, your body can be like a coach. It can tell you whether you should leave a situation, avoid a person or spend more time with them, whether you need an infusion of courage and confidence in order to get through something, or whether you have an injury or illness that needs your attention. It can get you back in touch with your natural sense of hunger and your natural instinct to move or to rest. It can answer your questions ("What do I need right now?") and give you advice ("I need to go to sleep").

You can use your interoception to discover things about your own body that you may never have noticed. For instance, can you tell which of your legs is stronger? Can you tell which side of your torso is naturally more lifted or pulled down? Are you sitting more heavily to one side? Can you discern in your own body by looking inside and using your inner sensors whether one of your hips is actually holding more tension than the other? Does this cause you to sit or stand unevenly? Are the muscles on one side of your body a little bit stronger? Are you always twisting just slightly to the left or right? Is one shoulder higher or lower than the other? If you focus internally, you can probably discover the answers to all these questions.

For many people, these imbalances are subtle but become more pronounced under stress. Stress can show up in the physical body as an exaggeration of imbalances that were already there, and over time, this can lead to pain or injury. Stress is something you can perceive internally when you tune in, and it's often most discernible through imbalance.

Let's say one side of your pelvis is stronger than the other side. When you're in a stressful situation, those strong muscles may take over and you may hold your body in a more extreme position, and if you do it for too long, that asymmetry of one side being more engaged than the other could cause your back muscles to spasm or a spinal disc to rupture. Before you know it, if you haven't been paying attention and adjusting accordingly, you're laid up on the couch in severe pain for a week or more.

PAIN

Pain is a teacher, and a loud call for introversion. The disconnected person will see pain as something separate that has invaded the body, but through introversion and being able to see connection, pain becomes a light that gets turned on to guide you. If you see pain as an invader, you try to extinguish it, whereas when you see it as a light, as a sign, you can explore how you might make a change.

I bet you've said something before like, "That's my bad knee." I say it, too, but I try not to, because that is an articulation of thinking of my body as separate from who I am. That is viewing the body almost inanimately, even though we know that it is fully alive.

Instead of saying, to use another example, "That's my bad shoulder," I try to say, "That's my teaching shoulder."

The body is not some baggage that is separate from us. Think of this perspective as a bridge to introverting physically. To do this, we can turn in and listen to the body. This is a method of communicating with ourselves. The body is a guide for navigation, and its guidance is always available to you. It signals with sensation, including pain. It talks to you with hunches, tingles, stomach turning, shivers, goosebumps, feelings of euphoria. It manifests your thoughts and emotions in all kinds of ways. However, it's just one side of an internal conversation. Instead of receiving these signals like they are a problem or even a punishment, introversion can be a pathway to receiving these bodily signals as guidance, or even as an alarm to wake up and change direction.

I don't want to minimize how traumatic and awful pain can be, and I certainly don't mean to imply that pain is "only" a signal. I do think pain is an important signal, but my hope is that if we can see pain as an indication of information, we can see it as a way to make use of the incredible intelligence of the human body.

My belief, and a lot of what I teach, is based on the presumption that there is a kind of intelligence intrinsic to the physical body. When something hurts, listen. Your body is trying to tell you something. In my own journey with pain, I learned (as many do) the hard way.

When I injured my knee in 1997, before I had ever taken a yoga class, I thought I had failed. Looking back, I now know my body was trying to tell me something, and I wasn't listening. Luckily, I had a friend say, "Hey, you should try yoga to heal your knee." In a way, the gift he gave me by encouraging me in that direction was a life-changing turn that started me on a path of learning to turn inward on my own.

Frankly, my yoga practice for many years was mostly extroverted. I wasn't really internally tuned in. There wasn't a lot of introversion. Not surprisingly, I got injured a lot in those first few years. Yet, every time I got an injury, pain nudged me to turn inward a little more. I got increasingly interested in exploring pain's source and finding ways to help my body heal. The more introverted my practice became, the healthier I got.

This is what sparked my interest in biomechanics, anatomy, and the physics of the body. I wanted to know and understand exactly what I was feeling, so I started to study with myriad teachers, as well as go to school, auto-didactically.

At the same time, primarily in my yoga practice, I spent years doing a sort of virtual inner dissection, like using a VR headset but with my own imagination. I explored internally, taking what I learned academically and applying it to what I was "seeing" and feeling inside. Admittedly, now when I get pain, my first impulse is still to think of it as a punishment, but I'm quicker to recognize that the pain is an indicator to change something. Now, one of my primary practices is introverting in response to pain.

It took a while before I began to see how I could do the same thing for other people. I started training with Desiree Rumbaugh, a teacher who was very focused on therapeutic alignment. I studied with some other teachers as well and also did a lot of my own research and reading. I studied books on kinesiology, especially the books by Doug Keller, who is a fairly well-known biomechanics yoga teacher. For seven years, I immersed myself in the world of therapeutics, biomechanics, and kinesiology. I even began to focus my meditations on healing and pain management. One of the greatest lessons from these teachers and my studies was how important it is to listen, and not just with my ears. The ability to sense energy is a kind of listening and a kind of physical introversion—it's listening with your ears and also with your entire body.

THAT BEING SAID . . .

Physical introversion, listening to your body, and making adjustments to your own postural patterns, isn't always enough. It's imperative, even if you believe in the power of your own body to heal itself, to not fall into the trap of forgetting to call upon professional help, like physical therapists and doctors, when needed.

In 2022, I sustained a back injury. This was the first time in fifteen years that I'd had an injury I couldn't deal with myself, via the therapeutics I had learned from my teachers. In other words, I couldn't get myself out of pain. I did my normal therapeutic work for a couple of days, but it got worse. That's when I decided I needed help, and fortunately, I had an incredible physical therapist who knew what to do for that injury.

The bigger point here is that introversion and interoception—listening to your own body—does not guarantee that you already have the answers to the questions that you pose internally. If you are a practiced yogi and you really know your body, you might know what to do when you have discomfort or even pain signals. If you don't, or even if you're not sure, it's probably smart to call upon a professional sooner rather than later. No matter the case, I encourage you to get better at listening, while remembering that none of us knows it all, and some problems require the intervention of a professional.

One of my favorite illustrations and one of the ways that I first became familiar with these ideas was because of something that happened with one of my students. I always used to start all of my yoga classes with a chant, and every once in a while, there would be someone with a great voice in the class. There was a young woman who often took my class, who had the most gorgeous singing voice. I love beautiful singing so I was always happy to see (and hear) her in my class. But then she stopped coming to class.

When I ran into her a few months later, I found out why. She told me that she got hurt in one of my classes. I was heartbroken that I could ever in any way be responsible for someone getting hurt, but I was so grateful that she was honest with me. It taught me a couple of really important lessons. One, I was doing the right thing in studying with those biomechanical masters because I needed to become better at listening to the physical cues, in order to teach a great yoga class. But almost more importantly, it taught me that as a teacher, the practice of simply enjoying beautiful singing in the way that I would at a performance—the pure extroversion of being an audience while I was the one in the seat of the teacher—was an abrogation of my responsibility and a giant missed opportunity to introvert and actually use the chant as a barometer for that present moment and what was going on with my students energetically.

I began to use the chant in just this way, during my classes, and sure enough, there was a correlation between the chant and the energy of the class. When the chant was generally off-key, dissonant, and un-unified, I learned to take that as a cue to be especially clear, succinct, and to spend a good amount of time at the beginning of the class creating unity. Conversely, when the chant was already pristine, I would take that as license to start a little faster and, while still paying attention, likely go a little further with the intensity and depth of the class.

Whether or not you consider yourself to be a teacher, this is something you can do, whatever your job or circumstance. Purely by introverting for a moment to feel the energy in the room, you may be better able to do your job, navigate your relationships, and help people who need your guidance.

My introversion practice had become a gateway into being able to actually heal my own injuries, or I should say, aligning my body such that my body is able to heal itself without always having to go to a doctor. That being said, I maintain that introversion can also help you to determine when seeing a doctor or other health professional is the best course of action. I'm not an expert on pain and I'm certainly not a doctor, so I can't tell you how to respond to the different things your body will tell you, but what I can say with devotion is that there is great benefit in learning to listen.

THE BREATH

The breath is the only thing that comes in and out of the body in a rhythmic way, day in and day out. Breath is a literal pulsation of introversion and extroversion. It's an energy exchange between the inner and outer you, between the world outside and the universe within, and of course also between the body and the mind. Bringing attention to the breath is a powerful tool for reversing the mind's attention and reminding you that the external world is not the only world. Where does the breath go when it goes inside? You can follow it in, follow it out, follow it in, and as you do this, you build a bridge between inner and outer.

Because of the rhythmic nature of the breath, it can be a remedy for anxiety, stress, burnout, or any form of mental dissonance. Just close your eyes and take a few deep breaths. There isn't anything more simple to us as humans than the breath. You could argue the heartbeat, but that has less of a voluntary component. It's harder to regulate. The movement of breath is much more under your control.

Even if you're stressed and your breath is either too rapid to find the pattern, or your exhales are much faster because you're in a state of crisis, you can regulate your breathing by paying attention to that rhythm, slowing down the exhale, taking a deeper breath. Even a minor level of regulation can put you into a calmer, more aware state.

QUICK T.I.P.

No matter why you feel a need to introvert, this T.I.P. can always be a way inside. It is the most basic, simple introversion you can do. It's just three breaths, but it could even be as simple as taking a single breath. You can do this with your eyes open or closed—certainly keep them open if you are in a situation where you need to watch where you are going. If you can stop and be safe somewhere, do this with your eyes closed. Closing your eyes has the benefit of being more of a visceral turn-in, since vision is generally directed outward.

1. Take a deep, slow breath in, not so slow that it feels like a struggle, but just a little more slowly and a little deeper than how you normally breathe.

2. Exhale slowly, rationing the breath to draw it out. Notice how it feels to breathe more slowly, compared to how you normally breathe.

3. Take another deep, slow inhale and exhale. As you do this, listen to your breath as if you are listening to a very important secret, so there is a quality to your listening that is introspective and goes beyond just observing. Give the sound of your breath your full attention.

4. Take one more deep, slow breath like this. Listen with intensity and fascination to the sound of your breath.

5. Now, consciously shift back to a normal rate and depth of breathing. Take a moment to reflect on whether those breaths shifted the way you feel. Reflection at the end isn't required, but sometimes, noticing a shift can crystallize and imprint the benefits of what you've done, as well as help to make it habitual, so you automatically turn to this practice when you have the feeling that you need it.

I've found for myself, and in most of the feedback I've gotten, that deep breathing is profound. People who have never tried taking deep breaths before are blown away by how catalytic it is for feeling better. Breathing doesn't fix the problem, it doesn't erase anxiety, but it gives you just enough space to feel like you're no longer past the threshold of agency. You can get to a place where you're just calm enough to be okay and recognize that you can either cope with or get out of a stressful situation.

Whether the asynchrony you are feeling is sped up, slowed down, or just off the beat, the rhythm of the breath and the rhythmic chanting of a mantra can help to restore that synchrony that can make you feel like you have a little more control over your situation. I think that's where we get the idea of counting sheep to fall asleep. I think it's why humans are so drawn to music. It's no wonder rhythm puts us back into a state of instinctual rightness. Counting, box breathing, and different kinds of breathwork with different ratios are all examples of how breathing can create resonance and synchronicity again (I'll explain all these techniques in chapter 7, where I'll also go more into the breath as a vehicle for introversion).

THE MIND

We so identify with our own minds that we tend to think that our thoughts define us, or even *are* us. But to believe you are only your mind is to believe that a part of you is the whole you. Your mind is just one part of you, and it can cause you a lot of grief—ruminating, obsessing, casting constantly into the past or into the future. It's a good thing we aren't only our minds!

We are least likely to feel like we can direct the mind when we are under stress. While stress is something we definitely feel in the body, it's also something we attribute to the mind. This is why people might say that your feelings are "all in your head." Stress may seem like it's "all in your head," when the day-to-day, mental noise of life leads us to overthink. It can be difficult to quiet the anxious mind. It can chatter like monkeys—there is even a term for the chattering mind, called "monkey mind." This constant mental noise can pull your attention in a direction that feels like inward, but which is really more of an extroversion because you are focused on the stresses of the external world.

Everyone knows what it feels like to worry, to be anxious, to be afraid, or to be in a position where you don't know what to do. We all know what it's like to feel like we lack the knowledge or agency to make a decision. We all know what it feels like to doubt ourselves, or to be so sure we are right that we can't really listen to someone else's opinion. We all know what it's like to criticize ourselves in our own minds.

But the mind can also be a spectacular vehicle for introversion because of its vast potential to take you absolutely anywhere. The mind can bridge the inner and outer, building a connection between your body and your consciousness. It can also build a connection between your mind with the mind of another, and you with everything outside of yourself.

Here's my favorite metaphor for the mind. Imagine you are swimming in an ocean in the middle of a squall. It's hard to stay above water, but your survival instinct tells you that you have to keep swimming. You might try to swim in one direction or another, but when you're caught up in all those turbulent waves, it can feel impossible to get anywhere. You can't control what the waves are doing. You can't control the ocean! You can feel like you're drowning.

But you have another option. You can take a break from the turbulent surface by going underwater, just for a moment. This is what it is to introvert the mind. It is the realization that, no matter what is happening on the choppy surface, beneath that surface you will find quiet and stillness.

This is introversion of the mind.

When you introvert, you know the waves (the external world) are up there, but you're getting a little moment of peace—a break from the struggle of trying to stay afloat and figure out how to navigate. Things settle. It's a different perspective. There, below the surface, you may be able to see a little better how to get to calmer seas. Your way out may become clear because you can finally see where you're going—you can gain perspicacity. Think about how much ocean there is compared to just the miasma of the surface. It's a lot bigger underneath.

You could argue that to introvert is always to use the mind, and that meditation is one of the most effective ways to introvert the mind intentionally. I'll talk more about more traditional modes of meditation in chapter 8.

THE EGO

Psychologists often divide the mind into different parts, and the ego is the part that extroverts. The ego is the part of the mind that resists introversion. We can't get rid of it in this life, but we can learn to manage it. The best way that I can explain the ego is to say that without the ego, we would walk into traffic. It is our external consciousness. Our "me-ness."

In psychological terms, the ego is generally defined as the personality—the outward you that you show to the world. It's the you that interacts with people, that gets offended or triggered, that is in a good mood or in a bad mood. When people describe you, they are typically describing your ego.

More simply, the word "ego" just means "I," as in, "I am Ross."

The ego is also sometimes described as the thing that makes us individuals and different from others. "I am Ross, so I am not Chris." You are you, which means you are not your partner, or your sibling, or your best friend. You are you because you have an ego. That's fine. It's necessary. It's how we distinguish ourselves and each other. It's a mode for separation, but as you know by now, there is value in separation.

However, if you overly identify with what makes you different from others to the point of being unable to find connection, that is when the ego becomes problematic. Yet, letting go of the ego is letting go of your identity. I try not to say that popular catchphrase "Let go of your ego," because I don't think it's possible.

I recently read one of those "Top 10 Things to Do" lists on Instagram, and one of the items on the list was, "Kill the ego." The idea of the ego is out there in the zeitgeist right now but the idea was that it's wholly bad. I think on a deeper spiritual level, that's a dangerous attitude. If a thing you're trying to achieve is unreachable (like "killing the ego"), you are striving for something impossible. You've failed before you begin.

Another one of my favorite words is defenestration. It's a word that comes from the Latin word *fenestra*, which means window. Defenestration is to throw something out the window, literally and figuratively. It's like throwing the baby out with the bathwater.

Oftentimes in a spiritual practice, people defenestrate the concept of the ego and I've always felt that was counterproductive. Yes, you don't want it to be the most important thing because that's annoying and can feel shallow. However, I don't think the opposite is true either, which is that there's nothing good or valuable about the ego. Over-identifying with your ego or having no identity at all are not the only choices.

It's true that the ego can be the source of arrogance, of narcissism, or more innocently, of trying to distinguish yourself, or be the best (like my competitive nature—that's egoic for sure). Putting the ego in charge without any inner direction or boundaries is oppressive to the heart. When the ego is in charge of the workings of the mind, then the mind is in a box. It can have trouble recognizing how much more there is to think about than who we are in the world. If you are all ego, it might make you famous, but it probably won't make you happy.

Yet, the ego can actually be a great navigator, and as resistant as it may be to introversion, the ego can be used as a vehicle for introversion. The ego builds a bridge between our deepest impulses and our socially appropriate projections. A conscious use of the ego for external purposes and an ability to put the ego in its place when it's not needed can help you build a bridge between your egoic projections and your inner self.

I imagine the ego as the one holding the map when you have to drive through life. Sometimes, that deep inner you, that complex spiritual you, needs to retreat and take a nap in the back seat while the ego drives. At other times, the ego needs to take a back seat and be quiet. When it comes to the ego, I would say, *Let go of the ego just enough, and soften what you keep just enough that it's not making bad decisions on your behalf, and allows you room to turn inward.*

SELF-AWARENESS

Introversion largely comes down to self-awareness. When you make note of your emotions, either in the moment or later, or even when you are contemplating your intention, introverting those moments by looking for a deeper perspective or a deeper meaning can take your introversion to the next level. To introvert is to turn in, but introverting your introversion means to turn in to a deeper level of intuition, wisdom, and understanding.

Let's say your feelings get hurt. Instead of just turning in and noticing the sadness that comes with your feelings of getting hurt, shifting to a deeper level can help you to detach from the situation, step back, and get curious about what happened. Moving beyond the hurt feelings, you can ask, *What is this really about? Why are my feelings hurt? Did I think I needed validation in that moment and I didn't get it? Was my ego hurt because someone criticized me? Was I hurt because someone said no to my idea? Was this really a reason to feel hurt? Can I accept my hurt and move on?*

This is where the wider perspective becomes valuable. You can take what you learn when you go deep inside and apply it back out into the world, moving on from the hurt feelings, or the anger, irritation, or impulse to do or say something to get even or hurt someone back.

THAT BEING SAID . . .

Self-reflection is great for understanding your own behavior and the behavior of others, but there is a point when too much self-reflection can cross over into obsessive behavior or can turn into an overly critical cycle of self-judgment. Just as with introversion and extroversion, it's the balance that counts. You can balance extroverted participation with introverted reflection, but you don't need to reflect constantly, or second-guess everything you do and say. Remember to feel dissonance versus resonance. If your introversions begin to feel dissonant, it may be time to go the other direction again.

You can also deepen contemplation about your intentions. Let's say you're working on a project at work, and the obvious goal is to just finish the job. You could introvert to notice that you are proud of your work. Or, you could go deeper and contemplate what it is about your work that makes you feel fulfilled. Is it that you have an innate desire to do things well? That you're providing for your family? That you're changing the world? That you love to exercise your creativity? Whatever it is that gives you satisfaction from work can become even more meaningful through introversion, when it becomes a deepener.

ANYTIME, ANYWHERE, ANYTHING

We can divide up what can help us introvert, but I also want to be really clear that no matter how I might separate things in this book (mind and body, inhale and exhale, introversion and extroversion), I want to end this chapter by saying that you can really make just about anything into an introversion.

Introversion begins with noticing, refining your ability to detect when you're extroverting or where your attention is focused, inwardly or outwardly, and more specifically to notice when you feel off or stuck or when you are in a moment where there's a problem. It can be just as important to notice when you're in a good moment, as a way of invoking gratitude and the recognition that you're stringing together positive, affirmative moments in life. That's a way introversion can elevate self-esteem, happiness, and contentment.

As you refine your ability to notice which way your attention is turning, and as you refine your capacity to discern your momentum in any given direction, you can continually ask yourself which way you are moving. Are you moving in an affirmative direction?

Are you in a moment you'd like to remember and cultivate by introverting? Or are you moving in a direction that feels negative, diminishing, defensive, and you want to introvert to change direction or get a new perspective? Are you feeling the urge to introvert because you feel stuck in a pattern you'd like to change? From that heightened awareness, you can apply the tools and methods of turning inward in any of a thousand ways—anytime, anywhere, through anything.

Truly, you can introvert in any moment. All you need to do is pause, and consciously take a deep breath. Sometimes I've felt that more magic can happen in pausing and taking a deep breath than in a thirty-minute meditation that borders on the psychedelic. At a deeper, more sophisticated level, that could look like pausing, taking a deep breath, and in that deep breath, opening up to the mysterious capacity and potential to reboot, start fresh, and look inside to the vastness that even in one breath can give rise to the solution that you're looking for, or the energetic shift that can transform a situation.

You can introvert anywhere because you take your introversion power with you everywhere you go. It's impossible for you to be somewhere without it. You know that anxiety you have when you've left your phone somewhere or lost your keys? You never have to worry about feeling that about the power of your inner wisdom. So whether you're at work, in transit, on vacation, in a familiar place, in a foreign place, all the benefits of introversion are available to you.

Whenever you find that you're purely extroverting in a situation— you feel little if any inner awareness of the experience, or you're in a rut, or you're moving really fast—you can take a moment of recognition that this would be a good time for introversion. Whatever it is that you're perceiving in that moment, whatever is in your field of vision or whatever you're hearing or whatever you're touching, you can use it to introvert by imagining how you are connected to it. Is it literally outside you? Of course. But a momentary practice of tracing a line connecting you to that external thing could result in a potentially catalytic transformational practice, in any setting you want to transform (because you want to change it) or imprint (because you want to remember it).

For example, your connection with a situation you want to change, such as a confrontation with someone, could completely change if you take a moment to imagine a line connecting you to that person, heart to heart.

Not only can you introvert anytime, anywhere, but anything outside of you can become a vehicle for introversion. Anything and everything you see, touch, sense, is already ultimately being experienced internally. You need only observe this. All of our extroversions have within them some degree of introverting because we perceive everything through the filter of our interior consciousness. That is the embodied, human mode of processing, understanding, and experiencing.

As you go into the practices in this book, remember that one of the main reasons we extrovert is that we use it to navigate life. We divide, label, categorize, define, identify, and separate because it feels safe to know what things are. But really, if you want to know what it's all for, good luck trying to find the answers through extroversion. It's like the old joke from *Hitchhiker's Guide to the Galaxy*: What's the meaning of life? 42. Of course that's absurd and there is no single answer, but that won't keep us from longing for one. There is something magical about the idea of all meaning fitting neatly into one perfect little box tied up with a bow. If only the answer really were "42"!

Meaning is too gigantic to reduce to a single answer. The big cultural, philosophical paradigms like virtue and how to be a good person and how to live your best life and how to be happy are complex, nuanced ideas that will never be fully described or understood in short, refined, "perfect" ways. The best we can do, as we move through the human experience, is to try to find the harmony that happens in the space between extroversion and introversion, each moving into and out of the other in order to place us where we are. Our deft flow from inner to outer in all the various forms, from the personal to the global, opens the gateway for peace, joy, and love.

T.I.P.

If you are experiencing something you want to remember, you can visualize a literal connection between you and that thing in order to imprint it. Whatever it is you are seeing, hearing, or sensing, imagine a shimmering golden cord connecting you to the thing you want to remember. For example, if you are looking at something beautiful, visualize that golden cord extending from that thing—a flower, the moon, a painting, or an experience with someone—into your heart. We tend to remember best that with which we have an emotional connection. Visualizing that connection as a literal cord can add emotion, presence, and value to the experience so you will remember it. As you do this, make a mental note about how it feels to envision this connection between you and something outside of yourself.

CHAPTER 5

INTROVERSION
IN DAILY LIFE

There are so many ways to introvert, so many ways to look within to connect the inner and outer selves and the self with the other, that I could never put them all into one book. But there are basics, from the quotidian to the esoteric, that I think you will find useful. The next few chapters of this book are meant to be a buffet of introversion tools. Read it in order, flip around and browse, or just start by choosing something that looks interesting to you.

I've got conduits for introversion, in-the-moment introversions you can use during the day, super-quick introversions you can use whenever you need to feel more grounded or get some wisdom from within, and introversions for specific pain points you want to address, like anxiety, anger, irritation, and that feeling you're in a despair spiral. I've also got breathwork techniques, yoga guidance, and information about more traditional forms of meditation and how to set up a regular meditation practice.

You can start easy or jump forward to the more traditional practices. There are no wrong choices. It all depends on who you are, where you are in your own practice, and what you seek. Once you try some of these, the touchstone is always: Did that move me towards freedom, or away from it?

My purpose in these offerings is to make introversion as accessible as possible to you, so I've taken many of the things people do throughout the day, out of necessity or just because they enjoy them, and attached an introversion practice to them. Not everyone keeps a journal or likes to write, but many (including myself) love to write down our thoughts, so let's start with how you can introvert by putting pen to paper (or hands to keyboard).

INTROVERSION THROUGH WRITING

If you're having trouble just sitting still and trying to go inside, writing can be a way in. Whether you write a lot of emails or write a blog or write published books, or you just write in a journal that nobody else will read, writing, especially habitually, can be a bridge to unveiling and crystallizing your inner wisdom.

If you are a creative writer or like to journal your stream of consciousness, you may find it easier to introvert. You may already think of writing as tapping into some higher source of creativity. Still, introverted writing—going within and letting the words flow naturally through you onto the page—can reveal the unshackled source of the person you present on the page. Let yourself be yourself as you write, without judgment, and see what comes out.

Writing for someone else—such as for publication or even an email—can feel much different. Writing for someone else is, by definition, an extroverted practice, compared to something like writing in a journal, but really, every time you write anything, you can introvert to make your writing clearer, more impactful, more interesting, and especially, more you. You may be much more likely to employ your logical faculties because your priority is to convey information, but even when you do this—even when for you, writing is a presentation more than an introversion—taking a moment to introvert first can make what you write more illuminative.

QUICK T.I.P.

As you write, stay present and immersed as the words come through. This can bridge the external and internal selves in a way that can make your writing more honest, more authentic, and more effectively communicative. Let yourself be present, even in your emails, and people will notice. Your writing will be more engaging and true. Introversion, I believe, really is the secret to good writing. (That and, of course, going back and proofreading before you hit "send"!)

Also, a regular writing practice, such as in a journal, can help you to get better at building that bridge between the inner you that feels something and the outer you that wants to convey information. The more you write, the wider and more transversable the bridge becomes, and the better you will get. People often find that their writing improves when they introvert as they write.

For that and many other reasons, I recommend journaling as an introversion practice, especially if you enjoy it. If you allow yourself to write freely in a journal without the fear that someone else might judge your writing, you give yourself the space and freedom to let your inner wisdom emerge. If you can think about that source as your inexhaustible, indefatigable, even omniscient mystical self, then what you write becomes a dialogue, from the inside out.

T.I.P.

One exercise you might try is to write down a question that has been gnawing at you. Maybe it is something like, "Should I find another job?" or "Should I go back to school?" or something more personal like, "Is this relationship worth saving?" or "How can I help my friend?" Then, just start writing, without thinking through it first. Let it flow and see what comes up. Think of it as you having a conversation with your higher self. You may find that you can answer your own question.

INTROVERSION THROUGH SPEAKING

Writing and speaking can both be modes of presentation. The difference is that speaking is almost always essentially extroverted. However, as with writing, introversion before and even while speaking publicly can make your words more powerful, more connective, and more essentially you.

Public speaking is an obvious presentation, but even a conversation with a friend is a kind of presentation. We don't all have to speak publicly, but as a teacher, it is something I do almost daily. Teachers, lecturers, preachers, salespeople, people who have to give presentations at work, and any other type of public speaking can benefit from introversion. You may not think you are a public speaker, but if you do Zoom calls, guess what: you are a public speaker.

Introverting while speaking in public can make your words sound (and be) more authentic, and more moving for your audience, than if you speak rotely or read from a script. To do this, think about your speaking, not as a lecture or a sermon or an exposition, but as a dialogue with yourself. As you speak, stay actively involved and engaged with what you are saying, rather than just reciting. When you bring awareness to your words as you speak them, responding to your audience as well as your own inner instincts in real time to adjust what you say and how you say it, you will give your words more power and impact. You will be in active relationship with your words, in real time. Some people do this naturally, but I think most of us can get better at it.

This is something you can do, and notice, not just in public speaking but in everyday conversation. I notice the contrast, or the binary, of speaking in an opaque, blocked way, versus speaking in an open and flow-state way, when I'm in Italy. When I speak to one of my students, trying to get better at Italian, I know I'll see them again so I get embarrassed about how I'm speaking. I hesitate, I pull back, I get fearful about the repercussions of making mistakes or making a bad impression, so I default to what I think I am most comfortable with, which limits my vocabulary and makes me less creative in what I say. I feel a separation between what I want to say and how I say it. However, when I get into a cab and talk to the cab driver in Italian, suddenly it's much easier. That relationship is a totally transactional relationship with no pressure, and suddenly I can speak Italian better because the fear goes away. I don't feel embarrassed. I'm never going to see this cab driver again. My vocabulary gets better, my conjugations get better, and my expression gets more interesting and creative. If I make a mistake, it doesn't matter so much to me. When I realized I do this, I began to try to bring that sense of freedom and courage into all my Italian conversations. It's not easy—the fear is still there—but it's getting easier to learn how to speak better.

T.I.P.

Can you rewrite your rote? Think of something you do over and over in your job or life. It can be an event, a task, or even just a rote moment, like brushing your teeth. The next time you do this, see if you can introvert your attention, listen from the inside, and experience that task or moment from a different perspective or with a different intention. Can introversion give that moment, that thing you do so often without thinking, a more elevated place in your daily routine?

For instance, if you have a staff meeting at the beginning of your day or week, can you use that meeting, not as a perfunctory checking-the-box experience that is usually the purpose of the staff meeting, but more like a barometer to help you either raise your game or sensitize your tone? Introverting in a situation like this can transform an obligatory, burdensome task or part of your job or day into a guidepost for how to navigate the next moment, or the rest of your day. Can you feel in your body the difference when you introvert? Try not to just listen with your ears but also with your body in that rote moment, almost in the same way your body can detect the difference between hot and cold. Can you sense what others might need from you? Can you sense the difference between "I need to inspire" and "I need to nourish"? How does that change your rote moment, and how does that newly non-rote moment change your day?

As a teacher, I've also noticed how an inner dialogue can enliven my classes and help me to be in the moment of teaching, rather than just reciting the standard script for the class I've planned. Interestingly, I've found that introversion has two different effects, depending on whether I'm teaching on camera without students in the room, and teaching on camera when students are also in the room. In some ways, the separation that the camera creates makes teaching easier because I can introvert more and be more internally conscious of how I'm teaching, without the energy of other students in the room. I can almost be more vulnerable and open. The camera becomes a bridge rather than a barrier.

On the other hand, when students are in the room, I can more easily engage with the energy of the room, so my inner dialogue informs my teaching in a way that becomes more focused on connecting to what's actually going on in front of me. In that way, the presence of students becomes a bridge that helps me to tap into my inner sense of what the class needs. The difference is fascinating to me, and I think both ways improve and potentially enhance my classes in different ways.

Introversion can help us to learn to self-remove the barriers and the separations that can keep us from trusting our communication and allowing it to be a bridge between what we mean to say inside and what we actually say in projection.

TECHNOLOGY NOTE

These days, it can feel like we all have on-camera jobs because of videoconferencing, or when we connect with family or friends who don't live nearby through video chats. Yet, most people don't know how to be on camera. It is a skill anyone can cultivate.

What I've found to be one of the big flaws of video conferencing is that people forget that they are in conversation. They keep talking without getting those subtle clues that it's time for someone else to talk. When you aren't in the room with someone, you may not feel the dynamic energy of conversation, if there is nobody to interrupt you. People are often afraid to interrupt others on Zoom calls because it seems more abrasive and aggressive to interrupt someone on camera, but without those natural interruptions, people can tend to go on too long. A lot of time gets wasted because they aren't getting those natural cues that it's someone else's turn to talk. As your introversion skills improve, notice how you improve in the extroversion of being on camera.

I think we have all had moments where we think back to something we said but wished we hadn't, or wished we would have said better, or thought but didn't say, or wish we would have thought of and said in the moment. Sometimes I think back to these moments and feel such regret for not saying what I thought about someone in the moment that would have been kind to say, or even not thinking of the clever comeback to someone who perhaps needed to be called out, or wish I would have been present enough to stand up for myself.

In fact, sometimes standing up for yourself, even being defensive, being forceful, refusing to be intimidated into silence, is the appropriate response in certain situations. When we don't speak truth to power, that is one of the best examples of how extroversion wins out over introversion. Introverting would be recognizing that you have a right to speak your mind, because ultimately you are just as valuable as the person who is trying to control or manipulate you or a situation. If you remember that in the moment, when you are faced with someone more powerful, that introversion can give you the courage to speak up.

As you speak, especially if you are nervous or don't feel confident, remember to stay engaged in your words. Let your inner self listen and contribute. Don't go on automatic pilot. Don't speak too quickly. Remind yourself that what you have to say is worthy, and doesn't have to be perfect. Surrender to the creative process and don't let the perfect be the enemy of the good. You don't have to be your best self when you go public—not even on that Zoom call. At the very least, you can try to draw from the deeper source of the person you present to the world.

QUICK T.I.P.

The next time you are talking to someone you trust, practice introverting to find the right words. Stay present and think about what you're going to say before you say it. Stay engaged, both internally and externally, to help you speak your truth but also recognize when it's appropriate to speak and when it's time to give the other person a turn. This can help you speak with more awareness, consideration, and a more mutual exchange of energy and ideas.

In this life, introversion will never erase the binaries of powerful and powerless, aggressiveness and defensiveness, or for that matter, clarity and opacity, but if it can get you a little closer to your own truth and doing what you believe is the right thing, then the practice of introversion is more than worthwhile—it's priceless.

INTROVERSION THROUGH STORYTELLING

Telling a story is basically the same as public speaking, but we all know some people who really put themselves into the story in a way that makes the story gripping, and some people whose stories are dull, or sound like rehearsed scripts, or who tell the same story over and over in exactly the same way.

A professional storyteller once gave me some advice about how to tell a story, and while she didn't use the word, essentially, what she said was that good storytellers introvert. She said that the best way to tell a story is to imagine, in the moment, as you tell it, that you are in the story.

For example, say I was telling you a story: "Once upon a time, there was a little girl who went on a journey, and on that journey she came across a bird." Okay, that's fine. But if I tell the story as if I *am* the little girl, the story becomes more animated and I become more invested in the telling: "Once upon a time, there was a little girl who, at just ten years old, decided she wanted to see the world. She packed up her bag and started out on what she imagined might be a fantastical journey. She wondered what she would see, as she crossed the road and went into the dark forest her mother always told her to avoid. She felt a thrill of danger and excitement, wondering what might happen next. Then she saw it: A brightly colored, magical bird, who cocked its head and looked down at her from a low tree branch.

The bird spoke!" Now, obviously I'm adding more detail, but making myself the little girl makes this easier to do because I'm in the story so it comes alive. If I'm the girl, I want to know why I'm going on the journey. I want to know where I'm going, and what it looks like. You hear me actually discovering the forest and seeing that bird as if I really did see it.

QUICK T.I.P.

The next time you are in a situation where you're telling a story, try living it, or reliving it, as you tell it. Don't just repeat the words. Imagine yourself in the story, as if you're narrating the story as it's happening to you. This is easier with stories that are true and actually happened to you in the past (I think this is part of why people love true stories so much—the teller speaks out of a place of knowing and engagement), but even if a story didn't happen to you or you're making it up, you can still put yourself into it. Something magical happens when you introvert to embody your own words. This builds a bridge between your interior world and the interior world of your listener. It builds a bridge between the past when the story happened and the present when you are telling it. It builds a bridge between the world of the lived experience and the world of the observed experience.

Another kind of storytelling is teaching, and one of the greatest teaching lessons I've ever learned from another teacher is to hear your own voice as you teach, and always to remember that you are teaching, not preaching (although the best preachers know that they are teachers). This applies to teachers as well as to anyone who is helping, guiding, or instructing someone how to do anything, whether that is working with a colleague, training a new employee, or teaching a friend how to knit or child how to do a cartwheel.

To do this, you have to go inside and listen to yourself and feel when to engage and when to instruct, when to ask questions and when to give examples, when the students are getting it or not getting it. Admittedly, this takes some practice, but you can start simply by using pauses. When you say something important, pause. Let the person you are teaching hear what you said, rather than rushing on. I think it's selfish and antithetical to the spirit of teaching, which is essentially service, if you don't give the student time to absorb the lesson. Otherwise it's just a performance.

This becomes even more important if what you are teaching is something that could potentially change someone else's life. If you run right over the important parts, you potentially steal a pivotal moment from the person who needs to hear what you're saying. You might not realize when to pause if you aren't introverting.

A few years ago, one of my students, who was attending a workshop I was teaching in Asia, asked me if I would mind speaking to her son, who was a senior in high school. She said, "You don't have to say anything in particular to him. I would just love for him to meet you." She asked if I would have coffee with him. I wasn't sure why she wanted him to meet me, but I agreed.

As soon as I began talking to him, I could tell he was brilliant. And sad. And a natural introvert. He was someone who went deep, mentally, but didn't have confidence. From what he told me, he felt lost and disconnected because he couldn't relate to other people and he felt like nobody understood him. He felt different than everyone else and didn't know how to fit in.

It was obvious from the way he spoke and the things he said that he was extremely intelligent. I told him that most of us feel different than other people in one way or another. Most of us feel disconnected, especially in high school, and feel like nobody gets us. And that's normal to feel that way. He would be okay if he just kept looking for people he could connect with. He would soon get to a stage in his life when he found the people who would understand and value him.

He might have to get used to the fact that not everyone saw the world the way he did, or understood things the way he did. He would probably need to learn to be generous in those moments, when people didn't understand him. I assured him that he would get better at reaching out, and would eventually find people to connect with. I told him, "Never let the people who don't get you stop you from being you."

Then I had a feeling I should shut up. It is sometimes my impulse to go on for too long, but I felt it was right to pause at that moment. We sat there together in silence for a little while.

I found out a year later, when I saw his mother again, that not only had her son been suicidal (she hadn't told me this before) but that something I said got through to him. This kid was someone who could go very deep within, but he needed the confidence to believe he would find a light down there. According to his mother, he made it through and he told her that our conversation made a difference.

I can't help thinking that the pause made a difference. If I had kept going on about something else, he might not have heard the part he most needed to hear. At the risk of an awkward silence in a tenuous situation, I ignored my controlling instinct to fill up the silence. Instead, I sat in silence with him, hoping he would absorb what I offered. Even though silence can sometimes feel uncomfortable, it's something we can heed and respect. Introverting as we talk to someone can help us sense when to let silence be.

I'm not telling this story to get any pats on the back, but to show that in this case, we were both introverting and benefited because of it. This conversation could have gone a lot of ways, but because of introversion, it went in a positive direction.

QUICK T.I.P.

The next time you are giving someone advice, hear your own words and see if you can cultivate an awareness of how the other person is receiving your words. Stopping to let someone contemplate something important you said to them can make the conversation more meaningful, as can remaining open to pause and absorb something someone says to you.

INTROVERSION THROUGH SERVICE

Service is ironically something you do for someone else externally that has the feel and effect of an introversion. Whether you do something small, like noticing when someone in your town is lost and helping them find their way, or something more extensive like volunteer work or commitment to a cause, find a way to do something for someone else even if it's as simple as holding a door open. It's easy here in New York because people are always lost—you can take your headphones off on the subway and notice someone who is confused and say, "Where are you trying to go?"

Service can be the remedy for finding connection when nothing else seems to work. Sometimes before I'm about to teach class, I feel a separation—I can get all up in my own head, either from nerves or because I really want to do a good job or because I know I didn't plan as much as I should have, or maybe I don't think my lesson is as clear as it could be, or maybe because something upsetting or stressful happened to me before class. I get into this complicated mental state of isolation and suddenly the red light is about to go on. That means we're filming, and I'm about to get up in front of the camera and teach a live meditation or yoga class in front of hundreds of people.

The thing that helps me to introvert and focus in a situation like this, that brings me towards a deeper, more grounded, more focused, more present place, is the idea of service. I've done this enough now that I can flip a switch and say to myself, *Be of service now*. This wipes the noise away, or at least pushes it out of the way temporarily, and lets me be deep in the flow of the moment.

Service can be like a skeleton key. There is great power in saying to yourself: *I am just going to serve*. I'm going to let go of my agenda. I'm going to do this. I'm going to do this purely for you, who's on the other side of me. This can be a very potent shift of intention.

INTROVERSION THROUGH STILLNESS

Sometimes, especially in the middle of chaos and upheaval, the most introverting thing you can do is to be still. Stillness can create an oasis in the middle of chaos. It can give you a chance to listen, to what someone else is saying, or to your inner wisdom, or just to silence, where you can begin to process your place in the chaos. This may be one of the easiest ways to introvert. Just stop. Get quiet. Hold perfectly still and see what happens. As with practicing silence, it can take courage to be still in the middle of chaos, but it can also be a transformative introversion.

For me, a moment of stillness was once so powerful that it became the moment I truly fell in love with my husband. It started when we went to see the ballet of *Romeo and Juliet*, choreographed by Kenneth MacMillan, score by Sergei Prokofiev. We had been dating for a while. At the time, Chris was a ballet choreographer (he's now also a two-time Tony-winning Broadway director/choreographer). Before I met him, I hadn't seen much ballet and had yet to know enough to discern what was good and what wasn't.

This ballet, however, even to my newbie eyes, was truly amazing. One thing that stood out to me was a moment in the third act when Juliet is in her bedroom after Paris leaves. She is in despair because she knows she is going to be married off to Paris. The score in this moment is magnificent and rapturous. I imagine that most choreographers would make use of this beautiful music with equally powerful steps. Instead, MacMillan chose to have her seated on the end of a giant bed, upstage, in complete stillness. It seemed antithetical to the music, but brilliant. And just as I was thinking this, Chris leaned over and whispered to me how masterful this was.

A few weeks later, we went to see one of Chris's ballets. In it, there was a similar stillness moment. At the peak of the music's intensity, the dancer stopped moving and held completely still. I was on the edge of my seat. It was like Juliet's stillness. There was something so powerful, so courageous, so life-changing in that moment, and I was hit with the realization that Chris understood in a way that surprised and thrilled me, that sometimes when everything is in chaos around you, what you really need is to be in stillness. His wisdom to choreograph stillness is more yogic than anything I've probably ever taught. In that moment, I realized his genius and his depth, and I felt closer to him than I had ever felt to anyone.

The power of stillness, for me, is undeniable. The hard part is remembering the magic of stillness when we're so often inclined to move, act, or fill the silence. There is so much power in just holding space. When someone you love is experiencing something traumatic or has had a loss, sometimes the best thing is to just be with them in silence and hold space.

INTROVERSION THROUGH ART

One of my favorite ways to introvert is by using music, theater, or visual art. I find these can be great catalysts for introversion because they were created by others who were experiencing inspiration moments. I think some of that rubs off, somehow. The Latin word "inspiration" is *inspiratus*, which means to breathe into, and it used to hold the meaning of divinity breathing into a person. When I'm in the presence of any kind of great art, I think about this—what inspiration was breathed into the artist to create this work of art, and what inspiration gets breathed into me when I experience it? Breathing consciously while in the presence of great art can put you in synch with what you are experiencing, and being in the presence of something beautiful builds a bridge from the everyday world to something ineffable or transcendent.

T.I.P.

I do one of my favorite introversion practices when I go to see a performance at the theater, especially if a friend is performing or if it's a show my husband has created. Right before the play, the musical, the opera, or the ballet starts, there is a moment before the curtain goes up when I do a quick eyes-open introversion. I set an intention to be open to the experience. I think something like, *May I be open to something I don't yet know. May I experience something I've never felt.*

You could do this before anything special you're about to do or witness—it could be a performance where you are in the audience, from your kid's school play to a concert to a baseball game to a Broadway show. You could do this before you're about to go to an art exhibit, or watch the sun set, or before you go on a date. Whatever it is, this little pre-event or pre-experience introversion can help you to get the most out of what you're about to witness or do, not because you are turning in and ignoring what's going on outside of yourself, but because you are turning in to be absorbed by what's happening outside of yourself. It's a simple reminder to be present and connected. You can do all this in under thirty seconds—just as the curtain is about to go up, just as you are about to walk down the aisle, just as you are about to step into a great adventure.

1. Make a mental note of where you are and what you are about to see or do.
2. Close your eyes and take a few deep breaths.
3. Tell yourself to be as open as you can. Especially if you're feeling stressed, breathe through the stress and try to let it go so you can be in the moment.

4. Imagine you're a child, full of wonder, ready to see something for the first time. Think about what you're about to experience with a bright optimism and hope.

5. Consider how fortunate you are to be doing what you're doing, and what an honor it is to be exactly where you are right now. Imagine your heart filling with gratitude.

6. Say to yourself: *I will absorb as much beauty as I can.*

I hope that at this point, you are fully realizing how, as I said at the end of the last chapter, anything and everything can be a source for introversion. Anything inspiring, anything challenging, any part of you, any part of anything outside of you, can lead you inward, if you use it that way. Now let's get into the many different situations where you can use introversion to intervene when you most need it.

T.I.P.

Imagine your interior landscape is a big room or outdoor space with nothing in it. Sit quietly with your eyes closed and imagine entering this room. How will you decorate it to represent who you are? If you are in a room, imagine creating the most beautiful or fantastical environment you can think of, that represents you, your aspirations, your dreams, your deepest longings, your preferences, your taste—anything that makes you feel like *yes, this is home.* What kind of furniture would you put in it? What color would you paint it? What's the floor made of? What do you hang on the walls? Or, if you're imagining an outdoor space, think about where you would put trees, or water, or flowers. Where can you see the sky, and where is the shade and shelter? Decorate your room, or your garden, but also remember that you can change anything at any time as you change. If you enjoy this introversion, repeat it regularly and update your personal interior landscape in any way that matches your current mood, needs, or desires.

CHAPTER 6

SITUATIONAL
INTROVERSIONS

ometimes, specific situations can call for introversions—your
inner wisdom is always there, and when you need to call on it,
introversion is the way, but how you introvert can vary according to
what's happening outside of you and how you feel about it.

Although there are many variations here, a structure that can be
useful when you introvert in response to a stressful situation (or even
a joyful situation) is to:

1. Pause.
2. Breathe.
3. Turn inward.
4. Ask yourself: *What do I need right now?*
5. Breathe and listen for an answer.
6. Ask yourself: *How can I get what I need?*

7. Breathe and listen for an answer. You might be surprised at what comes up, but whatever it is, think about it and see if it feels like freedom and fills you with a sense of calm or joy.

Know that you won't necessarily or always get a clear answer to either of the questions, but you may get an inkling, a sense, an intuition, or at least a direction to start moving in. I always ask myself: *What direction feels like freedom?* Remember that you have an infinite source of wisdom within. That's what you're tapping into when you introvert. Asking a question can help you to home in on at least a feeling of what to do next.

Here are some situations where you will likely find introversion useful. You can probably think of many more, but consider these scenarios and see if you can expand your own ideas about when and where you can most profitably introvert.

WHEN YOU NEED TO ASK FOR SOMETHING

For some reason, many people find it really difficult to ask for something they need or want. Introversion can help you feel more comfortable doing this because it can bring clarity around the what and the why.

If the thing you need or want is something someone else can give you—a job, a promotion, more time together, more time alone, help in resolving a problem—then I will say that it takes courage to ask. Introverting can help you build your courage. Imagine yourself asking for what you want. Think about the ways you might say it. Keep it in your mind, and then, be brave. Let your higher self guide you and infuse you with the courage you need to articulate what you want.

QUICK T.I.P.

This quick introversion can help you to find and access courage from within. Although courage can sometimes arise spontaneously, it's easier to access when you summon it with intention.

1. Sit or lie down comfortably in a safe environment where you can close your eyes for about five minutes.

2. Place your right hand on your lap or knee with the palm facing up and open. This is a symbol of openness and empathy.

3. Form your left hand into a fist, and hold your fist over your heart. Think of this fist as representing inner strength, boldness, and fearlessness. It is the power of standing up for yourself and your beliefs.

4. Take a deep breath, exhale, then feel your breath moving in and out. Gently extend your exhales so they are longer than your inhales.

5. Contemplate how strength and boldness coupled with openness and empathy are the keys to benevolent courage.

6. When you are ready, take a deep breath in, exhale fully, open your eyes, and move forward with a renewed sense of fortitude, power, and courage to do what you need to do for yourself and others.

Let's say you've really been wanting to bring up an issue with your boss that involves your success or happiness at work, but you don't think you are in a place to demand anything, or you assume or fear you won't be taken seriously. Maybe you worry you won't be able to express how you really feel, or that it's not appropriate to speak up, or that your boss doesn't get you. Whatever the objections to being honest and open and real, you are full of excuses.

Just turning in for a few minutes throughout the day can help you to develop an internal faith in your own light and power. Pause. Breathe. What do you need? How can you get what you need? Think outside the box, and then let your introversions and your connection to your inner fortitude help you to build courage, get clarity around the details, and develop a compassionate toughness in your approach that can help you feel more confident.

Then one day (it could be soon, or it could take awhile), you find you can just walk into your boss's office and you say what you need to say. Even if you don't say it perfectly, even if you stumble, you have achieved a victory by integrating your inner and outer selves in a way that authentically acts out in the external world what your inner self desires. That in itself is an integration that can make you feel better. And if you don't get what you wanted, regroup, and don't give up. Let your introversions access your inner creativity to find another way in.

WHEN YOU NEED TO SAY "I'M SORRY"

This is a tough one for many people, especially when the ego gets involved. Let's say you and your partner got into a big fight and you're both stubbornly holding a grudge or giving each other the silent treatment. Taking some time to turn inward and think about what happened in a more neutral way can help you to see if (1) you were actually wrong, (2) neither of you are technically wrong but you just differ in your approach, or (3) you are totally right but weren't kind about it.

Often, the way to connect is simply to apologize. But that's tough. Not only does the ego rebel against admitting being wrong, but it can feel vulnerable, and scary, to apologize. It can feel like you are giving someone else the power. This can take some courage, but if you can take someone's hand, look them in the eyes, and say, "I'm really sorry," that can completely turn a situation around.

If you can't sincerely apologize, or you really aren't sorry, but you still want to repair the connection, simply offer to listen without reacting or contradicting. Sometimes, all someone needs is to be heard, even if it doesn't solve their problem. It can be a silent way to open to what someone else is experiencing, and to them, it can feel as good as if not better than an apology.

In any of these scenarios, introversion can help you get to the place where you have the courage and strength to be vulnerable and say you are sorry, instead of letting your ego lead with, "You're wrong, I'm right." It takes courage to realize you'll be okay if you speak up, or apologize and let go of the need to prove you are right. It takes courage to let go of the satiation of being right in favor of the fortitude to actually turn the page and see that you are in this together and it's best to move on. It's Relationships 101—would you rather be right, or happy? It's one thing to have that question as a metric in your life, but it's a whole other thing to have the fortitude to do it when the shit really hits the fan.

If you don't have a way to go inside and tap into that fortitude, chances are you won't repair the rift. Likely, one of two things will happen: either you will force the issue and remain arrogant in your righteousness (defaulting to ego) but cause damage to the relationship, or you'll move on without actually facing it and being okay with it (defaulting to repression), and it's going to come out later, probably in a worse form. Just try turning inward to see in which direction your inner wisdom guides you.

T.I.P.

Sometimes it's hard to introvert at the height of emotion. After a fight with your partner, friend, coworker, kid, whoever, it could take a day or two, or even a week or more, before you're able to have a real introversion moment, and that's okay. You might need to spend some time feeling justifiably angry or self-righteous. But maybe the next time you have a fight, you can introvert in a day, and maybe the next time, you'll turn inside after ten minutes. Move closer and closer to the moment. Sometimes, you might move further away, and that's okay, too. Just try to notice that there is often a gap between feeling or experience, and recognition or reflection. When you are ready, try these simple steps:

1. Close your eyes and take a deep breath. Let it out slowly. Do this a few times until you feel calm.
2. Imagine the person you are having an issue with standing in front of you. Just look at that person, and imagine that person just looking at you, neutrally, neither of you speaking.
3. Imagine that the person in front of you begins to glow with a gentle, luminous light. Imagine you also begin to glow with that same gentle, luminous light.

4. Now imagine the glow of that person expanding, wider and wider. Notice that the light coming from you is also expanding.

5. When the glow surrounding the other person meets the glow surrounding you, imagine that the edges shimmer and form a connection between the two of you, from heart to heart.

6. Stay here for a moment, visualizing that glow that envelops you both, and that shimmering connection between your hearts.

7. Slowly let the image fade. Take one more deep breath, in and out.

8. Notice if you feel any different about that person. Do you feel ready to reach out? If not, you can try this introversion again, as many times as it takes for you to let go of your anger and feel that light-infused connection that exists between you.

WHEN YOU'RE IRRITATED WITH SOMEONE

If your partner, a friend, or a coworker is really getting on your nerves, or if you are in a situation where you are feeling peevish, a surprising question to ask yourself when you introvert is, *What do I need?* You might think that you're irritated because of someone else's needs that you find annoying or uncalled for, but often, irritation is actually based in something you need, rather than in something the other person is doing or some external situation. They might be triggering you, but why? This is what you can go inside to explore.

Often, what irritates people the most about someone else is to see or experience a quality that they have themselves. What is it about that other person that feels so triggering? Go inside and think about what it is exactly that bothers you. If you can pinpoint it, ask yourself: *Is this something I do?* If the person talks too much, are you irritated because you just want someone to listen to you? Maybe it's not the fact that they talk a lot, but that they are talking instead of listening, and *you* need a chance to talk. Is it because they did something rude? Personally, I hate it when people are rude. But whenever this bothers me about someone, I ask myself: *Am I rude?* I don't think so because I try extremely hard to be courteous, but if I really think about it, I can think of some examples... Maybe my irritation is about seeing what I have done played out in front of me in someone else.

Irritation could also be caused by something that bothers you from your past. You may get really irritated when you are criticized because a parent always criticized you. It's become a hot-button for you and you can realize, by introverting, that you may be overreacting. That was then, this is now.

All of this is easier said than done, and can take some deep examination of your own motives and qualities, but it can be fascinating to dive into your own mind and try to figure out what pushes your buttons and why—so fascinating that you might forget all about what that other person was doing that so irritated you.

If you're still irritated? Maybe you just need to take a deep breathing break, or do a quick centering yoga pose, or search inside yourself for some empathy, or practice service and ask the person who is annoying you: "How can I help?" Service is often a great way to dispel tension. Or maybe you just need to leave the situation for a while, to slow the momentum and regroup. Or, try this quick exercise to help you feel more connection with someone else.

T.I.P.

One of the binaries we all experience is the binary of you and someone else—the whole idea of individuals is a separation. This quick meditation is a way to bridge that separation.

1. When you are out in public somewhere, take off your headphones (or not), or do whatever you can to minimize distractions—this will depend on what you find distracting.

2. Look around and find someone that is a different demographic than you—maybe a generation older or younger, maybe a different gender or someone who simply looks or acts very different than you.

3. Mentally say to yourself, *I have a dream, and they have a dream.*

4. Think of what one of your dreams is. For example, *One of my dreams is to have grandkids*, or *One of my dreams is to travel to Japan*, or *One of my dreams is to learn how to paint.*

5. Look at the person who seems different than you and make up a dream for them, such as: *They have a dream to become a concert pianist*, or *They have a dream to go skydiving*, or *They have a dream to write their memoir.*

6. Finally, say: *We both have dreams.* Let this create a bridge in your mind between you and that other person.

WHEN YOU'RE ABOUT TO EXPERIENCE
SOMETHING IMPORTANT

Whether you're about to witness something beautiful (a sunset, an art exhibit), or something meaningful (your best friend's award ceremony, your child's graduation), or participate in something you want to remember forever (your wedding, the trip of a lifetime), you can introvert to cement the experience in your memory and heart.

Introversion can be an effective way to remember a joyful or beautiful experience. People often say, for example, that they don't remember their own weddings. Everything goes so quickly, and you're the center of attention. That can be so distracting and stressful that you forget to pay attention. Introversion can help you to recognize that you are in a beautiful experience. It can help you take it all in, so you don't miss it.

In fact, introverting to imprint and crystallize positive experiences has a cumulative effect. One of the long-term benefits of introversion as a habit is that as you do it regularly, you are weaving the tapestry or stringing the pearls on a strand that is your life. The more you imprint, the more you weave, the more pearls you string, the more you create your character, your very being. You are literally creating who you are by consciously weaving the tapestry or stringing together the pearls in the way you want to live.

This can get a bit mystical, but there is a kind of 1 + 1 = 3 theory that when you bring more conscious awareness to your life in this way, the universe begins to conspire with you. As you weave your tapestry with intention and a commitment to see the value and remember the moments of meaning, good fortune seems to happen. Things start to go your way more often. I think this is a mysterious element having to do with being in tune with something higher. As you begin to live with more consciousness and intention, notice if all of a sudden the subway is there right when you walk in, or you begin to find the things you lost more easily, or are given the things you need just as you need them. Notice if good luck begins to become the norm in your life. Is it because you're simply seeing the good more, or is it because you're internally synchronizing with your environment? I can't claim to understand it, but it is something I've experienced and witnessed.

WHEN YOU'RE PROVOKED

Introverting can be really useful when you feel off, unclear, sad, angry, or just out of the flow state in general. It's especially useful if you're being provoked or triggered. Introversion can help you determine how the authentic you will react to a provocation, rather than how your projected self might react.

I was provoked recently when I was traveling (although, by the way, travel is a great way to build more bridges). Our plane landed, and as soon as the "fasten seatbelts" light went off, I stood up with my bag and waited my turn to deplane—as one does. Everyone knows you aren't supposed to go down the aisle until everyone else seated ahead of you has gone first. There is an order to these things. But on this flight, someone pushed ahead and got off the plane without letting the people in front get off first.

I felt myself getting angry. Rudeness in general is one of my pet peeves, but I get especially irritated when people cut in line, and deplaning is a kind of line. I almost said something—I wanted to snap at this person and say, "Hey, dude, it's not your turn!" But just before I said something snarky, I recognized what was happening. In that moment, I turned inward. What did I know of this person's situation? Nothing. What was I assuming about this person? A lot. I asked myself the question: *Am I moving towards empathy and unity, or towards separation and negativity?* I took a deep breath and felt the bridge opening. Had I not been working on this for so many years, I probably would have gotten into some sort of altercation. Having those tools to introvert in the moment kept me from blowing up the bridge between external me and wiser, calmer, more judicious internal me. I deplaned feeling calm rather than angry.

This could apply to any situation where someone else's behavior bothers you, like getting cut off in traffic, someone stealing your parking spot at the grocery store, or someone in line ahead of you causing a long delay or a problem. When you can move towards empathy and away from a negative feeling of separation or righteous indignation, you may be able to transcend the trigger.

QUICK T.I.P.

It can seem almost impossible to introvert when you're feeling agitated or angry. To help you find a space from which you can act with more reason and wisdom, try this calming introversion.

1. Sit down somewhere safe where you can close your eyes. Put your palms face down on your knees. This is considered to be a calming hand position.
2. Breathe normally for a few breaths, then take a deep breath in.
3. Exhale to a count of 5-4-3-2-1.

4. Inhale deeply, then slow your count a bit as you exhale: 5-4-3-2-1.

5. Inhale deeply again, then slow your count even more as you exhale: 5-4-3-2-1.

6. One last time, inhale deeply, then slow your count yet again as you exhale, one more time: 5-4-3-2-1.

7. Slowly bring your breathing back to a normal, regular pace.

8. Open your eyes and notice how you feel.

WHEN YOU HAVE ACTED SMALL

A few years ago, I was doing a level 2 yoga teacher training. We were getting a lot of advanced information during this training and it was going great. Everyone was loving the experience, except for one thing.

One of the people at the teacher training was a woman I knew pretty well through our circle of yoga teachers. She is a super-knowledgeable teacher and wasn't shy about asking challenging questions, which I normally love. We were on day four of the training, and invariably, every hour or two, she would ask a question that wasn't really a question. It was a show-off. You probably know what I mean, when someone in a group wants to talk just to show off what they know.

I found it really disruptive. Every time she did it, I felt a little more frustrated and angry. I had the urge to call out what she was doing in a way that might shut down her behavior, but I turned in for a moment and played out how that would probably go. I realized this was not a time or place to lash out, so instead, I knelt down and softened my voice so I didn't sound angry or like I was mansplaining. I said, "What was your actual question?"

But, even in a lowered-body, soft-voiced way, it came out sounding pedantic. No matter how soft my voice and nonaggressive my physical stance, I was pointing out to everybody, in the form of a question, that she wasn't really asking a question. And it caused a big problem.

I thought it was over and done with, but there was blowback and major drama after class that we all had to deal with. I had turned inward, or so I thought, but apparently not enough because while I recognized and modified any extroverted signals of potential meanness, the condescension in my choice of words was still discernible to everyone. What I didn't see in the moment was that I only displayed the trappings of kindness, without any of the truth of kindness. Had I introverted just a little longer or a little deeper, I might have recognized this.

Interestingly, later I made a point of connecting with her to repair things and we became friends. She's a coach, so I asked her to give me a coaching session. What better way to learn what she was about? This was one of the most valuable things I think I've ever learned. She pointed out in that moment, "Small Ross took over, and could have been bigger." Now I have a little image in my head when I sense Small Ross coming out—I think of it as Little Napoleon Ross—and I find a better way around the problem. It makes me introvert and think, *You're about to do that thing. Choose something better.*

Through your introverting, you will become more self-aware of your behavior when you extrovert, and if you discover parts you don't like, parts of yourself that act in a way that doesn't feel like your best self—maybe it's Small You—you can set up a mental alarm bell to alert you when that side of you is starting to emerge. Are you acting from a place of communal empathetic awareness and service, or a place of ego that makes you feel vengeful? It can look like exactly the same thing, but you feel the difference and other people feel the difference, too—I've found the human bullshit detector is one of our superpowers.

T.I.P.

Look back at moments when you know you weren't your best self. What was the cause? What were you doing? What insecurity might have been lurking beneath? This introversion can help you to cleanse that feeling, forgive yourself, and move forward with a higher consciousness of how you want to project yourself in this life.

1. Envision yourself in a situation when you don't feel good about your behavior.

2. Don't think about what you did, but instead, recall how you felt in the situation. See if you can embody that feeling again.

3. As you do this, take a deep breath in and imagine the air rising up through the center of your body in a column.

4. Then, take a long slow exhale, imagining the breath like a waterfall, pouring warmly from the crown of your head to the soles of your feet, letting the breath wash away your sense of smallness so you can open up to your higher self.

5. Repeat until you feel calm.

WHEN YOU'RE HAVING A BAD DAY

We all have bad days, but they don't have to stay bad days all day long. When things aren't going right, or you're making mistakes, or it's just one of those days when you feel dissonant or off for no apparent reason, introversion can help you to reset. Remember that when you feel dissonance, you can begin by recognizing that feeling, then finding the value in it, and then introverting to build a bridge to a different state or direction.

Begin by taking a moment to turn inside and feel your feelings. What are they right now? Can you label them? Are you irritable? Self-righteous? Insecure? Afraid? Angry? Anxious? Tired? Hungry? Just identifying the feeling could present the answer to your problem. Maybe you just need to take a nap or eat something, or calm down. However, if you can't place it and it simply feels like dissonance or asynchrony, it can help to find a rhythm. Do a few sun salutations, if you regularly do yoga. Listen to music with a dominant beat. Better yet, dance to the music, or play some music if you play an instrument. Or sing. Or, try this introversion, which uses rhythm to shift you from a dissonant to a synchronous state.

T.I.P.

To restore a sense of synchrony and resonance to your day, try this exercise, which taps into the natural pulsation of your heartbeat.

1. Sit comfortably in an upright position, or lie down comfortably, in a quiet place.
2. Take a few calming breaths.

3. Put your right hand over your heart, then put your left hand over your right hand.

4. Close your eyes and feel your breath moving in and out.

5. Can you feel your heartbeat beneath your hands, or hear the beat of your pulse in any part of your body? You may not be able to feel or hear it at first, but if you settle in and really focus on trying to feel or hear it, sometimes you will be able to.

6. If you can feel or hear that internal beat, concentrate intensely on it for a minute or two. If you can, synch your breathing to it, such as inhaling for five beats, exhaling for five beats.

7. If you can't actually feel or hear it, tap your left hand over your right hand in the beat that you imagine as your heartbeat—tap TAP, tap TAP, tap TAP. Do this for a minute or two, focusing on the regularity of the rhythm.

8. Slowly bring your hands to your sides and notice if you feel any difference—calmer, more in synch, more in tune with your environment.

WHEN YOU LOSE SOMETHING

Think how many times in life you've lost something. Whether you lost your keys, lost your luggage, lost a job, lost a friend, loss is almost always somewhere on the pain spectrum between discomforting and traumatic. This goes back to our human nature and need to connect. When we lose anything, we can feel bereft and disconnected, even for something trivial.

One way to approach dealing with loss is to tap into your sense that everything is connected. If you believe that, it means you aren't just connected to everything inside your perception, but also to everything outside your perception. So when you lose something, you only lose it on the personal level or the surface level (not to diminish the notion of surface—it doesn't mean inconsequential). When something is no longer a part of your life, introverting to find a unity perspective is in a way allowing the thing you lost to be there still, even if it's in an imperceptible form.

This of course does not take away the pain of loss. It might diminish it, just to feel that somewhere, somehow, that thing (or person) is still connected to you, but more likely it's simply going to steady you enough to begin the process of healing, calling upon hope and courage, or simply in the case of material items, realizing that you might not miss that thing you lost as much as you think you do. You might be able to replace it with something better.

In the case of friendships or relationships, their loss is almost never easy, but part of what you can contemplate as you introvert is whether you can find access to a kind of sage generosity, with which you can tap into your ability to trust that the relationship or friendship ran its course—that everything has a beginning and an ending. Even though you may in the moment wish with all your might for that person to be back, for the relationship to keep going, you can step into the part of you that trusts you'll be okay. You might not in that moment be fully able to see the potential, but perhaps you can trust that it's there when you're ready.

And remember: Introversion is not necessarily about solving the problem or fully taking away discomfort. It's about mitigating the stress and anchoring us in a place where we can make better choices or move forward.

QUICK T.I.P.

Next time you leave your phone somewhere, or you can't find your car keys, and that initial anxiety grabs a hold of you, pause, take a deep breath, and say to yourself, *I acknowledge that I'm anxious because I misplaced my [keys/phone]*, and then say to yourself, *If I don't find them, I'll be okay*. Then, you may be in a better frame of mind to do the work of either looking, or figuring out how you're going to handle whatever is in front of you without them.

INTROVERSION FOR MORE TRAUMATIC LOSS OR WHEN SOMEONE YOU LOVE DIES

Loss when you lose an item or move to a different home is one thing, but when someone dies who was close to you, or you lose someone in some other way, like through a divorce or a break-up or even a child growing up and moving out, something that was outside of you passes through you and takes you to a new place. You can feel lost and alone, or overwhelmed by grief. You don't really know what happens after death—all you know is that the person who was part of your life is now gone.

This is not always the time to introvert. Trauma and grief, according to professionals I've learned from, can require some space and time. Remember, it can be important to just let yourself feel what your body is trying to feel.

Death in particular can also trigger a kind of deep spiritual experience. If you experience the death of someone, it can be hard to accept that they are no longer in the human realm, and your grief can make you feel as if your very soul is shifting. I think part of the reason why death feels so extreme to us is that we tend to deny that we're going to die. We know rationally that we will, but we don't like to talk about it or even think about it, and death is a huge source of fear for many people.

I see this in the yoga world all the time—there is this strange idea that if you do enough healthy things, somehow, you can put off death forever. Nobody says that in so many words, but people talk about how long they will live and how they might prevent getting any kind of disease.

Of course, you can't avoid death completely, but in your introversions, you can contemplate death to get more comfortable with the concept. This can help you not only to accept that it's going to happen to you, but to be more accepting to the fact that it has happened to someone you love. If introversion reverses for a moment what we do most of the day, which is to extrovert, and if yoga puts the body in positions that balance the positions we hold our bodies in for most of the day, isn't death the ultimate way to do the opposite of what we do every day? We live, and the opposite of that is we die. Contemplating death takes us out of the navigable, binary, time-and-space realm, and that is beyond human understanding, but we can surmise that it might be the ultimate state of unity—the wave falling back into the ocean.

Once you're in a place where introverting feels right, another kind of introversion beyond contemplation is to place the mystery of your loss inside the mystery of your vast inner self. In the case of the passing of a beloved friend or companion, imagine them within your own heart. With loss and trauma, it's incredibly important to remember that introversion isn't a cure. It's a salve, a bridge, ballast. And it can be a connector.

WHEN YOU NEED TO FEEL GROUNDED

When life gets stressful, it can feel like you're floating and can't quite get your feet back on the ground, metaphorically. This can feel confusing, dizzying, and like you are unmoored and adrift. I used to feel ungrounded a lot, and how I helped myself feel more grounded when I felt like things were spinning out of control was to actually, literally, physically feel a solid connection between myself and the ground.

QUICK T.I.P.

To feel more grounded in the moment, if you are able, go outside and stand, sit, or place your feet on the actual earth: on grass, dirt, sand, rock, or whatever surface you can find where it's acceptable to be there.

Begin by taking a solid position, with both feet flat on the ground. Imagine that gravity has suddenly made everything much heavier, so much so that it's hard to move. Send all your energy down into your feet, even down into the earth, anchoring you in your body and on the planet itself. Stay there until you begin to feel more connected with your physical body and surroundings.

A great way to feel grounded is to get out into nature. Take your shoes off and walk or just rest your bare feet on the grass, the dirt, or on a beach or in a park that's accessible for you. You can also sit or lie down on the ground. Breathe and feel the planet beneath you, supporting your weight, holding you safely.

T.I.P.

Another way I like to feel more grounded on my commute is to "surf" on the train. If riding a train or subway is part of your normal routine—or on those rare occasions when you might ride a train or even an airport tram—you might try this. Only do this if you have good balance and make sure you are safe, near a bar or railing, or something else you can hold on to if necessary.

As the train begins to move, bend your knees slightly and don't hold on to anything unless you begin to feel unsteady. Move with the train and feel the tracks beneath you. Shift your weight as the train shifts so you remain balanced, as if you're on a surfboard, surfing along the track.

This exercise attunes you to the train and to your environment because you must introvert to focus solely on balancing as you hurtle forward. (But again, please do this safely! Always have a bar to grab. You can even lean your body against the bar slightly, if that makes this exercise more accessible.)

You can also do a version of this when you're a passenger in a car. (Don't try this while driving.) The vibrations of a car move through the entire vehicle including into you, so you can become aware of this tire-to-road contact and feel like you are grounding as you are moving.

WHEN YOU NEED A NEW PERSPECTIVE

There is a category of meditation called perspective-shifting meditations that can help you introvert in order to see a situation in a different way. Whatever it is that you recognize you need to see differently—maybe it's something you don't like but have to accept—think about the first time astronauts saw the earth from above. This completely shifted how they viewed and felt about the earth. Even when the rest of us got those photos back, it was paradigmatically different to visualize the world for the first time as it really is. We saw the earth not just as a globe but how it really looks. Through most of human history, we weren't able to do that. We could only imagine what our planet looked like. Now, we know because we were actually able to view it.

This is what I think about when I need to change my perspective. The astronauts literally rose above the earth, but you can rise above a situation metaphorically in order to change how you see things. I think it's a bit of an extroverted introversion, to imagine yourself hovering above a situation to see how it looks. How would it look if you were watching a fight between you and your partner from above? Imagine you're looking at a feed from a spy cam in the ceiling, or that you are an alien visiting from another planet, watching and wondering what these strange humans are doing... or relating and thinking, "Yeah, we act like that, too." It's a split-second introversion that could change your participation in the situation, in the moment.

QUICK T.I.P.

Rising above can be a gateway to detachment. Imagine that you are watching yourself from an elevated perspective, like from a hot air balloon. If you can separate yourself, even for a moment, from the perspective of personal involvement, you may be able to discover what someone else needs or feels. You may also gain insight about how your own behavior looks from the outside.

WHEN YOU'RE STUCK IN THE SHADOW

We can all get stuck in a negative state, sometimes short-lived, sometimes persistent. When you feel rooted in a sense of anger, sadness, frustration, discontent, despair, burnout, even rage and catastrophizing, it can be extremely difficult to see your way out of it.

One of the less stigmatized descriptions of "negative emotions" or emotional states that we instinctively want to get out of is "shadow states" or "shadow aspects." There is abundant literature from authors who are experts in psychological and sociological fields that explains the presence of and the work with this part of us, but the essence is that we all have a darker side.

Negative emotions are essentially deficit states. Something feels missing. They are not villainous. They are cloaks that can be removed, and the shadow cloak is usually heaviest when we feel like we don't have enough of something. We don't feel like we have enough freedom, or time, or willpower, or knowledge, or ability. And we definitely feel at a loss when there's an absence or a diminishment of love, superficial or profound. But it's in the wider view that we can see the absence of something as simply an absence, rather than seeing it as punishment or unfairness or bad luck.

To see negative emotions this way can be useful and can make introversion feel more accessible. Once we do find our way inside, and we're able to pause, take a breath, and step back from the myopic tension of the shadow, that's when we can start to use introversion to bring some light. What can start to happen then (maybe in the moment or depending upon the depth of the emotion, maybe over a period of time), is that we can change our relationship to the emotion from being its subject to becoming its sovereign. We can shift from the mindset of "this is happening to me" into the mindset of "how can I use this?"

THAT BEING SAID . . .

I want to acknowledge really clearly here that even for the most experienced meditator, or even if you've practiced introversion for a while, sometimes the shadow state persists. Before addressing how to introvert in these particular moments, I think it's worth saying again that sometimes introversion is not the highest choice. I've certainly been sad, angry, and scared, and needed to just sit in that state for a while. I didn't even want to shift out of that emotion. This is not my field of expertise, but I think it's important not to idealize introversion. It doesn't fix all problems, and I think we all need to be honest with each other when it comes to our deeply complex humanity.

Consider sadness. One way to navigate the shadow emotions related to sadness, once we've stepped back, is to introvert through a lens of gratitude. Think about what you feel is missing from your life that's causing your sadness. See if you can go within to recast the deficit as a gift. If it's something that you used to have that you're missing now, see if you can view it as a gift you received in the past. If it's something that you've never had, that you long for, then see if you can view the gift as aspiration and hope. Sadness may remain and in fact, there are some situations where it's inappropriate for sadness to ever fully go away. But as opposed to sadness in isolation, we can begin to transform regret to contentment and despair to hope.

What about anger? When it comes to anger in all its fiery forms, we can turn in to our inner courage and remember that we always have more fortitude than we think we do. We're usually angry when it feels like something has been taken from us, or on behalf of someone else we feel connected to (even if a stranger), when something has been taken from them.

As always, the first step is to pause, feel the anger as dissonance, find the value in it (is it calling for a change, for action, for forgiveness?), and shift to a unity perspective by building a bridge between anger and courage, patience, and the steadiness to rise above the cause of anger.

QUICK T.I.P.

"Rising above" can sound lofty, but it can be a useful practice for exploring your anger. Anger feels oppressive, like it's something above you, weighing you down. Going inside and imagining your anger as a fiery ball, then imagining yourself literally rising above the ball of anger and observing it below, can help you to step into a place of empowerment. Once you're more in charge, it's easier to choose to set anger aside or possibly see it as energy that gives you the fuel you need to take action.

We've all undoubtedly experienced shadow in the form of fear, insecurity, and anxiety, whether it's feeling lost, worrying about having enough, or being scared of what's ahead of you. Turning inward is a way of tapping into abundance consciousness, which is the opposite of fear consciousness.

I remember going on a vacation in Mexico a couple of years after having a smartphone. We were staying at an eco-resort with no electricity. Even though I'd been on silent retreats, in this situation I was shocked to learn that I wouldn't have any access to my devices. I had thought I would, so I hadn't had any time to prepare for this. I was angry but my primary emotions were anxiety and fear that I was going to miss out on a lot, and that I wasn't going to be able to accomplish the things I had planned to get done.

Admittedly, it took a few days, but since I couldn't do anything about it, eventually I realized I was going to be okay without those devices. Pretty quickly after that revelation, it was utterly joyful to be without them.

That's clearly an example of material or superficial fear, and fear is often much more existential. But turning inward, especially when you begin to do it more regularly, can give you the tools to face fear and insecurity with the deep truth that the power we have within is more than we'll ever need and more than we'll ever use.

In fact, many people throughout history who have been in grave danger or hazardous situations, or who have experienced tragedy, great misfortune, or horrific injustice, have gone on to create some of the most inspiring art, or have gone on to be living beacons of hope. No one can or should be expected to triumph in the face of tragedy, but the fact that so many have—the simple fact that humans are able to create such intensely meaningful beauty out of tragedy—is a testament to the deep capacity we all have to choose abundance, even in the most challenging circumstances.

All that being said, I want to be super clear: it's imperative that we respect the severity of emotional states like depression, abusive anger, and debilitating fear to the level that we never hesitate to seek out professional help. But for the more typical shadow moments, introversion can provide relief, and might even be the gateway to finding a transformational solution. Just like other introversion practices, recognition is still primary, but when it comes to emotional challenges, the work that you've done in widening the scope, the practices of turning inward to remember that there's always more than we're perceiving, that's the work that will really come into play in these difficult moments or stages of life.

T.I.P.

These specific introversions are surprisingly powerful for breaking out of the rut of a shadow emotion to find a wider or different perspective.

Quick Tip for Sadness

Pause, take a deep breath, and recall someone who taught you something or who helped you. Visualize them as if they were in front of you. Pretend you are holding a present that they will love, and you offer it to them as a symbol of abundance and gratitude.

Quick Tip for Anger

Pause, take a deep breath, and imagine a moment in your past when you or someone you know could have used some help. As an introversion of empowerment, imagine a version of you with superpowers shows up and saves the day.

Quick Tip for Fear

Pause, take a deep breath, and think of something in nature that amazes you. The vastness of the universe, the beauty of a perfect sunset, the vast ocean, the spare beauty of the desert, a lush forest, the variety of nature itself. As an introversion of wonder, abide for a few moments in awe of that image.

CHAPTER 7

INTROVERSION
AND YOGA

Even though this book is about the practice of introversion, I wanted to add a little bit about yoga, because many of my readers may know me from my yoga classes. To be clear, this is not a book about yoga. However, I've been teaching yoga and breathwork since 1999, so I do think it's appropriate to address how these practices can be powerful vehicles for introversion.

The word "yoga," which is most commonly translated into English as union or the yoking of at least two things, is widely used in different ways, often determined by context, geography, spiritual lineage, and understanding of the history and traditions of yoga. As yoga has become more mainstream, as a modality of fitness and wellness, many people think of yoga simply as the poses that are done in a flow-style or vinyasa yoga class.

Traditionally, however, "yoga" is a term and a concept that contains a multiplicity of practices, ethics, and philosophy. How we define yoga is an important conversation when it comes to honoring tradition and avoiding cultural appropriation, particularly given that Western cultures, which have helped promulgate the benefits of yoga, have also been the source of more colloquial and less fulsome understandings of the larger yoga tradition.

You may never find yourself in a situation where you have to define yoga, but since it is somewhat complex, and potentially a sensitive topic, it's a worthy contemplation, particularly if you find yourself going on to study more along these lines.

For me, like many things in my life, I try to find the value in the different definitions and uses of the word. There is a part of me that is a traditionalist, partly because I love history, and I've experienced the richness and depth that comes with learning about sources and lineages. In the same way that a student may compliment me by saying how a meditation helped them, I've made a point of always giving credit to my teachers. I think it's both honest and good for us to be readily able to credit the source of knowledge and wisdom we benefit from.

At the same time, I also have an arguably liberal perspective on the usage of the word "yoga." I know classes like "Yoga with Wine" are offensive to my friends who lean toward a more traditional definition of yoga, and I respect the importance of that perspective. However, I'm a believer in gateways. Even though I love the subtle and profound power of these practices now, I took my first yoga class for a purely physical reason. So for me at least, it was a nontraditional yoga class that started me down this path that made me the person I am today.

One way for you to employ the practices of introversion when it comes to determining your definition of yoga is to see it as one of the examples of the separation paradox. Yoga can be one thing and simultaneously many things. By turning inward, you can discern which facets of yoga hold value for you.

All of that being said, this is a book about looking within, not about the myriad aspects of the larger yoga tradition. I don't take you through any yoga poses in this book, but instead, approach yoga specifically in terms of how it can be an introversion practice. Luckily, there are hundreds of yoga classes of mine you can take on the Peloton app, if that's an interest you want to pursue. Or, obviously, there are many qualified yoga teachers out there who offer personal instruction.

I do want to go over some high-level aspects of breathwork and yoga as a way of illustrating how those two aspects of yoga are naturally suited for introversion. Breathwork blurs the line between inner and outer, since the breath moves in and out of the body, which is why it's one of the best vehicles for bridging the separation paradox and simultaneously a way to draw your attention inside.

Yoga poses are a great introversion bridge because they are static yet dynamic and therefore, they provide an opportunity to shift between external sensation and internal awareness. Because yoga uses the body in a way that is often opposite of how you use the body throughout the day, it can encourage you to turn inward to notice how the poses make your body feel.

Additionally, yoga poses often include breathwork direction because many of the poses are meant to be done in certain ways that synchronize the body with the breath—another bridge. We'll start with breathwork since breathing is something you've always done and will always do in this life. It's also on the short list of things we do involuntarily but that can also be done with more awareness, with boundaries and regulations. In the Ashtanga eight limbs of yoga, breathwork is one of the limbs, known in Sanskrit as *pranayama*. There is great literature on the history and practices of this ancient tradition.

From the very first quick turn-in, you've actually been doing breathwork. Simply pausing and taking a deep breath is a fantastic first step in experiencing the power of breathwork, and is equally a powerful gateway to introversion. Here are some ways to take your breathwork further.

BREATHWORK EXERCISES

Another way to think of the breath is that it's proof that we naturally shift between inner and outer—it's a built-in tool for introversion since it never stops going in and out. If you don't believe me, pick either an inhale or an exhale and see how long you can stick with just one. On a more serious note, simply becoming aware of the breath, even before you begin "controlling" it with exercises and regulations, can yield many of the benefits of deeper or more sustained introversions. In fact, sometimes, I've experienced a massive shift in perspective by stopping and taking three deep breaths, usually in a moment when that was the least obvious thing to do—in other words, usually when I was angry.

When you become conscious of your breath, even without changing anything about it, you can hook your attention to the breath. As you inhale, let your attention be drawn inside. As you exhale, let it flow naturally out again.

Or, you can alter your breath. You might take a deep breath and hold it for a few seconds as you bring your attention within and see how it feels inside of you as you hold your breath. Or you can listen to and focus on the nebulous space between breaths.

Becoming aware of your breathing is in itself introversion because you are focusing your attention on an internal process, and it's something you can do anywhere at any time, even if you just notice and feel your breath for a few seconds. However, you can be more systematic about your breathwork, turning it into a regular introversion practice that can have great benefits for stress relief and a feeling of calm and serenity.

For some people, breathwork is their main mode of introversion. You can make it a regular practice by starting and ending your day with a few moments of conscious breathing, or with breathing exercises like the ones that follow. Start with brief sessions, and work up to longer periods of breathwork to bookend your days, if you find it useful for you and you like doing it. You'll also see that in chapter 9, in the four-week introversion training program, I've integrated breathwork sessions that gradually increase in length.

There are many types of breathwork and they all have merit. Here are a few that you can practice. These are all good options for integrating into a daily introversion practice.

Box Breathing

Box breathing uses a 4-4-4-4 pattern. Each 4 represents a count, so in box breath, you will inhale for a count of four, hold your breath for a count of four, exhale for a count of four, then hold your breath again for a count of four. Traditionally, you would do this exercise sitting, as instructed below, but you can also do a few rounds in any situation where you need to calm down.

1. Sit comfortably with an upright spine, supporting yourself in a chair or with bolsters, blankets, or pillows, if you can't sit comfortably without support.
2. Bring your attention to your breath without changing it. Notice how it moves in and out of you.
3. Now, bring a structure to your breathing. Begin by inhaling slowly for a count of four, at approximately the speed of four seconds (it doesn't have to be exact).
4. At the top of the inhalation, hold your breath for four seconds.
5. Slowly exhale for four seconds. Exhale fully.
6. At the bottom of the exhale, hold your breath for four seconds.
7. Repeat four times, or go for as long as you like.

Mind-Body Breathing Meditation

The breath is a literal bridge between the outside and the inside of the body, and because it is naturally rhythmic, this meditation can help you to ease dissonance and feel more in tune with your environment as well as within your own body, helping to sync up your body and your mind. Read this through a few times so you can do it with your eyes closed. Or, read each step, pause and follow the instructions, then open your eyes and read the next step, proceeding through the exercise this way.

1. Find a comfortable sitting position, supported if you need it.

2. Sit up nice and tall so that you have a steadiness to your posture.

3. Soften your facial muscles and your shoulder so that there's a sweetness rather than a rigidity to your posture and how you feel.

4. Close your eyes and take a few deep breaths.

5. When you breathe in, see if you can feel like the breath is water. It's liquid. You're filling up with an inhale.

6. As you breathe out, think of the breath more as light rather than water. So you're exhaling in a luminous and spacious way. Do that a few times.

7. Now, when you breathe in, imagine your hips are a basin and let the liquid fill the basin first. Let the liquid rise up with your inhale until it reaches the crown of your head and begins to evaporate into a sparkly light.

8. Exhale and from the top down, emptying the light from the crown of your head, all the way down to the basin in your hips.

9. Do this for a few rounds, inhaling liquid to fill up from your base, exhaling light from the top down.

10. When you have a sense of calm and peace, slowly open your eyes, stretch, and readjust back to the external world.

Alternate Nostril Breathing

This is a traditional *pranayama* breathing exercise called *Nadi Shodhana*. This exercise creates a relationship and a rhythm between the binary of left and right by directing the breath through one side at a time, switching back and forth. This pranayama is often credited with bringing balance to the nervous system and it's a good exercise for synchronizing the body and mind when you're feeling off.

There are multiple ways to practice *Nadi Shodhana*. In the example below, you shift to the other side while briefly holding the top of the inhalation. As with all the exercises in this book, read it a few times through so you can do it with your eyes closed, or reach each step, pause, follow the instructions, then proceed to the next step.

1. Sit comfortably with an upright spine. Support yourself if necessary with bolsters, pillows, or blankets.

2. Breathe normally through both nostrils for a few breaths.

3. Fold the first and middle finger on your right hand into the thumb pad to give you better use of the tip of your thumb to block the right nostril, and the tips of the fourth and fifth fingers to block the left. (Blocking just below the hard cartilage of the nose is more effective than blocking the nostril opening.)

4. Hold your right hand in front of your nose, hovering over where you would block the nostrils.

5. Exhale your breath completely.

6. Softly block the right nostril with the tip of your thumb and inhale through the left nostril.

7. At the top of a full inhale, with almost imperceptible movement of your hand, unplug the right nostril and block the left nostril with the tips of your fourth and fifth fingers.

8. Exhale through the right nostril.

9. Keep the right side open for the next inhale.

10. Shift again at the top of the inhale, unplugging the left nostril and reblocking the right nostril to exhale through the left side.

11. Keep repeating this process, remembering to shift the blocking at the top of the inhale, ten to twenty rounds, depending upon your comfort level and experience.

Breathing Through

Another form of breathwork that helps to connect you to your environment is to breathe through things. I like to do this meditation while walking, especially in nature, but you can also do it sitting. In this exercise, you will imagine you have a sort of ethereal tube connected to either a close or far object. Breathe into it, then let it breathe into you.

Another way to do this is to breathe as if you are the thing you're looking at. If you are outside, you could anthropomorphize a tree, a bench, a flower, or anything you see. Pretend the thing you are looking at is breathing (even if it's an inanimate object). As you gaze at it, or walk by, sync your breathing to what you imagine that object's breath to be. If you see a frog, you might imagine, and embody, a fast pulsing breath. An old oak tree might have a long, slow, hissing breath. A flower might have a light, delicate breath, while a bee might have a vibration to its breath, which you could imitate by vocalizing a low hum.

QUICK T.I.P.

Pretend your breath is a song you love that you haven't heard for a long time. Whatever pace that song has, whatever depth it has, whatever volume, just listen extremely passively, like you're walking by a storefront and you catch the song on the radio or on a sound system from inside. Stop for a moment and just listen to your breath like a song you overhear.

If you want to explore breathwork, or learn more about prana-yama, look for a yoga teacher with experience in teaching pranayama, or look online for more breathing exercises that use different ratios and techniques. But remember, just slowing down your breathing and introverting for a few minutes is a powerful practice.

CHAPTER 8

GUESS WHAT?
YOU'RE MEDITATING

You might consider that you're getting pretty good at introverting by now, and perhaps you're wondering about a more traditional kind of meditation. There are certainly ancient techniques that have evolved or been adapted for modern use, and you can find some of these, as well as guidance for establishing a more structured or traditional-seeming practice, in these last three chapters. However, I'm still going to be a little stubborn in this chapter, even when I'm talking about traditional meditation.

There are of course a lot of traditional meditations that I advocate and I practice, but I'm intentionally going to keep it pretty straightforward and basic in this book, so as not to get too far away from the idea that turning inward can happen in many different ways—in fact in almost any way—besides traditional seated meditation. I never want to get pinned down by the word "meditation" or any particular definition of it that's narrower than "introversion." If going forward you ever use the word "meditation" to describe what you've learned from this book about introversion, and you're talking about something other than traditional seated meditation, and I heard you, I would say, "Cool. Well done."

My hesitation to get too specific is because this book really is not about meditation—or it is, but it also isn't. Again, I greatly respect and honor those who practice more traditional forms of meditation, and I again ask your forbearance because ultimately, even as I give you instructions, I hope you will remember that "meditation" really can be as simple as pausing and turning inward, even for a microsecond in a conversation, or pausing for a couple of moments during your workday. When you are doing something more traditional like a seated meditation, you are still pausing your day and creating an environment that is like an oasis or a sanctuary. You are still turning inward. You can choose to make it a little more sacred than the rest of the day, and safe enough also that you can close your eyes so the going inside isn't just metaphorical or subtle, with a literal shutting off of vision to add internal vision to internal attention.

But it's still turning inward.

That being said, I am going to give you some more structured versions of introversion or even traditional meditation practices, especially in week two in the four-week program for establishing an introversion habit, which is in the next chapter. I'll take you through using the breath as a vehicle to take your attention inward, along with visualizations, affirmations, or mantras, and employing some of the many traditional meditation methods of turning in. This is, I admit, where I cross a subtle threshold into my version of traditional meditation.

I think it's incredibly important for you to know your own power and capacity to supercharge your meditation practice with the idea that inside yourself, you already have and already know everything I have to tell you. You know how to introvert. As I've said many times before, you are already doing it. Just remember that even when I tell you how to do sitting meditation, you don't have to do it in any one particular way. You can sit if you want to, but you don't have to. You can stay still, or move and stretch. You can close your eyes, or open them. You can breathe through your nose, or through your mouth, or both.

My hope is that instead of you going through the years of frustration and seed planting I went through, I can help you do that work so you can experience that bridge and see the connections available to you just by turning in, in all its forms. You'll get there faster than I did.

MAKING INTROVERSION SPIRITUAL

One of the common views of traditional meditation is that meditation is only defined as a highly spiritual, seated practice that is characterized by illuminative, transformative, mystical experiences. Often, one of the things people say conversationally about what's expected is that meditation involves a cessation of all thought. There is a famous teaching in yoga that is often interpreted to mean that meditation success is only achieved when the thoughts stop.

I'm of the belief that both of those things might exist: the illuminative spiritual transformative moments, and the cessation of thought. However, in my experience, transformative moments in meditation are actually pretty rare. Personally, the majority of my meditations usually feel like just turning inward, often pedestrian and on good days, just utilitarian. And I gain great value from that. Every once in a while, I'll have a really powerful profound mystical experience, so I know they do exist, and I do believe other people who say they have experienced such things as well.

However, I'm of the belief that cessation of thought doesn't truly exist. Now, I could be wrong, but I look at it from a scientific standpoint. There are always energetic movement of synapses and neurons and electrical impulses in the brain, until the point that we die. So, even though you might experience a feeling of cessation, the thoughts perhaps slowing down so much that it feels like apparent stillness, the electrical impulses in the brain are still firing. I've gotten close to that feeling of mental stillness, and I understand why people are attracted to that idea. It's the opposite of the noise of the monkey mind. In no way am I diminishing the cessation of thought as an instinctual goal. But the reality is that something is always moving in there.

I believe that ultimate cessation is a little bit of a white whale. If you know the story of *Moby-Dick*, the tale is about how chasing the uncatchable is such a waste of a life. Should we have goals? Of course. But if we see the failure to reach those goals as an indication of our worth, we're probably getting in our own way on our spiritual journey.

I know I was getting in my own way. Because of my type-A personality and my self-criticism, meditation for me was at first an extroversion. It was something "other." I felt the pressure of doing it correctly, sitting in the right way, trying to achieve that cessation of thought, trying to achieve all the goals people associate with traditional meditation—inner peace, the ability to fully concentrate, enlightenment. I know I'm not the only one. A lot of people have a "should" mentality around meditation. They see it as this external thing they should be doing, and if they don't get the promised results, they think they must be doing it wrong.

THAT BEING SAID . . .

If you're in a community, or a class, or at a retreat where, for whatever valid reason, meditation needs to be defined as a particular style or type or result or technique, or you simply want to practice the more traditional form, I respect that as well. I myself practice sitting meditation, as well as other types of introversion. If the form you learned isn't even in this book, I hope you will consider that this book simply offers other ways to a similar, or to the same result.

I've told you how meditation completely changed for me when I began to think of it as introversion, and then as turning inward. The practice became much more fundamental than I had perceived meditation to be. Only then did I begin to get the feeling of actually introverting in my practice.

That being said, it's not that I was doing meditation wrong. I only thought I was. Even when I had a feeling of extroversion during meditation, I was planting seeds that would sprout later. I say all the time that you can't do it wrong, and I mean that. But what I felt was that I was missing something. When I had the revelation that meditation was just turning in, that gave me the perception to realize that oh, I can meditate, and it's not as hard as I thought it was. Even when you are using a more formal or traditional meditation technique, you can still demystify it by thinking of it as simply turning in.

SETTING UP YOUR SPACE

When I first started to get serious about meditation, I asked one of my long-time meditation teachers, Sally Kempton, for some advice. She suggested I make more of a ritual out of meditation. She understood that the structure was freeing. Putting some discipline around it, formalizing it, sanctifying it, was what worked for me at the time.

Formalizing a meditation practice is like putting a frame around a piece of art—that could mean scheduling it, using special props, or ritualizing it in any way. Elevating your meditation with ritual offers you the freedom to then experience it in your own way. For me, sitting meditation has become a thing that is a little more precious, and that catalyzed a very organic commitment and a gestation—I have grown spiritually since I've started meditating more formally and more regularly.

The first tip Sally Kempton gave me, to up my meditation game, was to shower before meditation. It's a bathing ritual. It signifies that what I'm about to do is important enough that I don't want to sit down in my normalness, in whatever I was before. It adds to the sacred and ritualistic nature of sitting meditation.

Second, I made a sacred area for meditating. You can meditate anywhere, of course, but if you have a space where you always go, that too adds to the ritualistic nature. It doesn't matter if it's a corner of a well-used room, or a room devoted to that purpose only. Here is how I suggest you prepare a meditation space.

- Put some effort into cleaning it really well, organizing it, and decluttering. It's a respect for the space where you will meditate.
- In that space, set up an area that is sometimes called a *puja*, for devotion. This can be a decorated corner or even a small altar on a low table you can sit in front of when you meditate. Cover it in a scarf or colorful fabric, or scatter flowers over it. Add pictures of people you love or revere, quotes that are meaningful to you, crystals, favorite pieces of jewelry, fresh flowers, pleasantly aromatic candles (be sure nothing will catch fire), figurines, pictures, or other objects that put you in a spiritual frame of mind. This is totally optional but many people enjoy doing this.
- Control the climate. If you can have either a heater or an AC unit running so the temperature is comfortable in the space, meditation will feel easier. If you get chilly easily, fold a blanket or shawl next to your altar, for use while meditating.
- Spread out a yoga mat for yoga practice, and a meditation cushion or enough blankets and pillows that you can sit comfortably. If you have other props, like yoga blocks, bolsters, or an eye pillow, bring those to your space.
- Prepare a space to sit comfortably.

HOW TO SIT FOR MEDITATION

There are several classic sitting positions for meditation, but in general, sit on the floor in a cross-legged position with a straight back, if this works for your body. Sit up on a cushion or folded blankets that raises the level of your hips to the level of your knees. If you have flexible hips and your knees actually fall closer to the ground in a cross-legged position, you don't need to sit as high. If you are less flexible and your knees are raised, sit higher. In either case, put something soft under your hips and your ankles so everything touching the ground is touching something soft and you feel comfortable and supported.

A PHYSICAL PRACTICE TO PREPARE FOR SEATED MEDITATION

This is a physical exercise to create a feeling of both groundedness and spaciousness inside the body. It can be a good exercise to do before you plan to sit in meditation or to spend some time in stillness while introverting. Try this on some days before you engage in a sitting practice and not on other days. Notice if it makes a difference, making it easier to sit, or possibly more difficult. It can also be a good practice to do before any activity where you want to feel open and present.

1. Stand up straight, feet a little less than hip distance apart, arms hanging loosely at your sides. Or, if you are unable to stand, sit with a straight spine as well as you are able, in a chair or on the floor.

2. Lean to your left side, so your body weight is centered on your left foot (or if sitting, on your left hip), almost but not quite balancing. The right foot (or hip) is on the ground or seat, but not holding much if any weight.

3. Put your hands on your hips, and push down on the left side of your pelvis. Imagine you are driving your foot (or hip) into the ground. Feel stability, groundedness, and safety as you imagine your foot (or hip) is heavy and immovably planted.

4. As you continue driving the left side downward, at the same time, imagine lifting the left side of your torso, from your waist to your forehead. Imagine all that energy moves upward until it pushes your left eyebrow up.

5. Feel the downward movement of energy from the pelvis, and the upward movement of energy from the waist to the eyebrow.

6. Now shift your weight to your right foot (or hip) and push down on the right side of your pelvis. Imagine your right foot (or hip) is driving heavily into the ground.

7. At the same time, lift the right side of your torso, from your waist to your forehead, making your right side so spacious that your right eyebrow raises.

8. Shift slowly back and forth until you have settled into the middle, with your weight equally distributed on both feet and over your pelvis.

9. Push down on both sides of your pelvis with your hands, imagining driving into the ground, as if your feet (or hips) are deeply planted. Feel the safety and security of this attachment to the earth.

10. At the same time, lift up from the waist to the crown of your head, feeling the energy moving upward until you feel like you could push on the ceiling with the crown of your head.

11. When you feel deeply grounded but also spacious and open, relax your body and prepare to sit for meditation—or move on with your day.

Some people use a classic setup of a padded flat cushion (a zabuton) with a round meditation cushion (a zafu) in the center on it, to raise the hips and have padding under the feet and knees. Some people like to use a meditation bench so they can sit with their legs under them, without actually sitting on their legs. There are many options—find something that feels comfortable to you.

THAT BEING SAID . . .

Comfort is important in meditation so pain isn't distracting you, pulling your mind outward when you're trying to turn inward. However, it's also beneficial to push just a bit past your own limitations. If your discomfort is more mental than physical, or you feel compelled to get up even though you are physically fine, see if you can push through it and sit a little longer than you think you can. In other words, physical comfort is primary, but don't be afraid to push the envelope of your own mental fortitude.

Once comfortably seated, rest your palms on your knees, face down or face up, or clasp your hands together and hold them in your lap. You can also put a cushion in your lap to rest your hands on if you need more support for your shoulders or wrists.

This is the classic setup. In reality, though, sitting on the floor without a backrest isn't comfortable for everyone and can be so uncomfortable that it makes meditation too difficult. It's totally fine to modify this position and still get just as much benefit out of meditation. If sitting upright is hard, you can sit against a wall. If you will be meditating for a long time, it's okay to sit in a comfortable chair. With practice, you may be able to move to the floor eventually. Sitting on the floor takes some getting used to, if you don't normally do it.

Unless you've been meditating for months or years, you may find that even when sitting on the floor is comfortable at first, at some point your hips and back will get tired and feel strained or your foot will fall asleep. When you feel discomfort, listen to that feedback from your body. It's fine to stretch out your legs, stretch your back, even stand up and stretch for a few minutes, move into a different position, or even lie down. There are no rules.

WHAT HAPPENS DURING SITTING MEDITATION

As you sit to meditate, the mind can seemingly get noisier and louder and more agitated when you close your eyes and try to sit still and go inside. Know that that's normal and there's nothing wrong when that happens. It's not an indication of flaw. Instead of vilifying it, give yourself some space to think, *There goes the monkey mind. There go all those thoughts.*

Even in the presence of monkey mind, you can still meditate. You can float apart from the thoughts and watch them. Think of them not as anything bad but as puppies on the playground. *You puppies, don't run away, just hang out over here in this nice playpen, and I'm going to meditate over here.* There are no unfriendly dogs in this dog park. There is no thought that will run rampant.

Then you can go into some breathwork, like box breathing (page 151), or focus on an image, or say a mantra, or just count your breaths up to ten, then start over. Every time you get distracted by the puppies, go back to your breathing when you realize you forgot what you were doing. Also, it's really fun to watch puppies play, so when you notice you're getting pulled back into the play, it's good to have breathing and meditation techniques that keep you anchored.

But don't worry if you get caught up in your thoughts. Remember, the point isn't to stop thinking. It's just to look within. If what you see within are thoughts, then you can watch those thoughts and see them with curiosity. You can listen to your body, to your mind, to your wisdom, or you can just breathe. Do what feels natural.

And if, as you sit there looking within, you feel a little nervous, that's natural, too. Even when you have the space to turn inward, to contemplate or to navigate a question or a problem, it can feel scary because you don't know what you're going to find in there. There is a lot we don't know about the mind, even scientifically. Unless you are a psychologist or a neuroscientist, you may have some trepidation around diving too deeply into the mind. It's no wonder so many people resist meditation.

But it's your mind, so really, there is nothing in there that isn't already you. Sometimes, it can help to visualize something. I've had multiple meditation teachers use the image of creating a tapestry or creating a string of luminous pearls, in the same way you collect a set of experiences in this life. You could visualize a calming scene, or focus on a single point like a flickering candle flame, or you could repeat a word or an affirmation and feel the sound of it inside your body. When in doubt, you can always come back to the breath—that bridge between the inner and outer you.

It can also be helpful to know that on some days meditation will feel better and on other days, it won't feel as good or as easy. That's normal, too. For example, on the day I wrote this, I was struggling to meditate. I didn't enjoy it, my concentration felt elusive, and I couldn't get to a place that I normally go. What usually works for me is to envision that there is this energetic force in charge of the universe, and I try to just go with it: *Take me away, I'm all yours!* But on this day, even that wasn't really working. I couldn't get into a good place. I had a couple of good moments but after thirty or forty minutes, I gave up.

In fact the whole day felt off, not just for me but for other people around me. Some days just feel crosscurrent. But, even if it wasn't the best meditation, not fun or joyful, I 100 percent believe that I'm navigating the off day better than I would have if I hadn't meditated. I would be blown away if it didn't make a difference. If I hadn't meditated, I believe my bad day would have been worse.

IS PRAYER THE SAME THING AS MEDITATION?

Prayer and meditation are alike in some ways and different in other ways. In my opinion, prayer and meditation are more alike than different, especially when you are in a place of longing, or sorrow, or you feel like you are isolated and can't break through into a state of connection. Sometimes, all you want to do is send a question in—or out. It depends on how you conceptualize it, but I think what matters more is that you are seeking connection, and that is an introversion. People often think of prayer in terms of asking for something profound, something needed. That is also often the focus of meditation. Ultimately, they can be the same, or they can be different, or they can be both. You decide.

Even when it doesn't feel great, even when you think you're doing it wrong, have some trust in your own spirit and capacity, and even in the mystery. We can't ever fully know what's happening in a meditation, but you can trust that you are planting seeds, and part of planting seeds is trusting that nature's going to do the work. There is something else involved besides your conscious, identifiable mind-body-spirit that makes those seeds bear their fruit. Be open and try not to judge the experience of meditation. Trust that there might be value in what you deem as a negative experience. There might be—in fact, there almost certainly will be—value later.

MAKING MEDITATION A ROUTINE

Whether or not you decide to meditate on a schedule in order to do it more consistently depends on who you are. If the last thing you need in life is more structure, you may benefit from playing around with meditation without having a lot of boundaries around it. It should be something you enjoy because it makes you feel good. Or, if you are more the kind of person who just wants someone to tell you what to do, and you know that unless something is more constructed and scheduled, you probably won't do it, then set up a program for yourself.

Once you start to notice a shift and you begin to see and feel the value in what you're doing, you can change the metric a little bit. You can start to build more of a practice, putting more parameters around it. Maybe you'll just sit quietly once a day, and once a week you will sit in meditation for ten minutes (using any of the short meditations or T.I.P.s in this book). Then you can continue to work up from there. Set a goal, like twenty minutes every morning, or don't. If you do set a goal, give yourself permission to take as long as is comfortable to get there. Try a quick one once a day, and once a week do something at a deeper level. After some time, maybe go longer, five to fifteen minutes. Maybe it will be a month down the line, or six months, or a year. Another goal could be to check out the Peloton app and try some of my classes, and classes from the other instructors, that are more organized and instructive than what you can do from a book. Or, you might decide to take a class somewhere in person, whether that's a yoga class or a meditation class or something else.

THAT BEING SAID . . .

One of the traps people can fall in when they try to make meditation into a routine is to think they "should" do it. When you get caught up in the "shoulds," you can begin to feel like meditation is a chore and you can begin to dread doing it. For some people, not being disciplined about meditation might encourage them to do it more. People tend to apply discipline to things they have to do, like going to work, while things they want to do, like going on vacation, don't require discipline. Especially when you first begin meditating, it can be more effective to do it only when you feel like doing it, and as the benefits start to accrue, that is when you might put more of a structure around it, because you want to, not because you "should."

QUICK T.I.P. REMINDERS

As with all introversion exercises, read each step, follow the instructions, then open your eyes to read the next step. After doing these exercises a few times, you probably won't need to look at the steps anymore. You could also have someone read the instructions for you, or even record yourself.

Sitting (or not): Generally, these introversions assume sitting with legs crossed in a vertical posture. However, you can *always* adjust your sitting position, take a break to stretch out your legs, stand up, lie down, or whatever you feel your body needs. It is 100 percent okay to be comfortable when you are doing any introversion practice! When you are sitting, support yourself with bolsters, cushions, blankets, pillows, or whatever you need. It's also okay to sit in a chair or lean against the wall. Shift your weight until you feel centered in the middle, with the crown of the head over your pelvis.

Eyes: Closing your eyes makes it easier to turn inward, but if you feel like you have to open your eyes at any point for any reason, that's completely fine. Just close them again when you feel ready.

Breathing: Another general rule about sitting in meditation is that breathing is through the nose, with mouth closed, but if this feels stressful to you, or if you are congested, it's totally fine to breathe through your mouth, for a moment, or for the whole introversion.

Guided words: These introversions are guided, but that doesn't mean you have to believe everything I say or always resonate with it. Let my words wash over you and, with a healthy skepticism, contemplate what feels right or real or true to you. And remember, you can always introvert without being guided by anyone's words.

Never forget that you can't do this wrong! Instead, radically embrace your experience, no matter what it is. Some days are simply easier than others, and that's natural and normal. What matters, or I should say what will really make changes in your life, is a regular practice of introversion.

MOVING MEDITATION

There is a misconception that you have to meditate while sitting. In fact, there's a tradition of walking meditation called *kinhin* that involves walking back and forth very slowly while meditating. I'll loosen up that definition even more. You can meditate (i.e., introvert) while running, dancing, lifting weights, and especially walking anywhere, as a mindfulness practice that still allows you to navigate through the real world. (A caution with any walking or running meditation: you could get into such a flow state that you won't notice you're about to step into traffic, so be sure you're walking in a safe place without uneven surfaces, like you might encounter in the woods, unless you're really paying attention to your environment with a mindfulness practice like the one that follows.)

Once you've set yourself up for a safe walk, you can fall into a rhythm with a mantra. A mantra is a word or set of words you repeat to focus the mind. I especially like the mantra "I am that," and then, "That is me" (this is *ham sa, so hum* in Sanskrit, which is a nice mantra to say, as long as you know what you are saying) to use with moving meditations. As you walk, be mindful of your surroundings, soaking in the beauty of the present moment. As you encounter "beings" along the way, direct your mantra to them.

You might walk by a tree that catches your attention. Imagine pulling the tree in, introverting the image by thinking, *I am that* (or *ham sa*). You are the tree. Then perhaps you see a deer, a squirrel, or a bird in the woods and you think, *That I am* or *That is me* (or *so hum*). The tree, the deer, the squirrel, the bird—they are all you and you are them. This mantra is about connection. As you flow back and forth between what is within and what is without, you can find the unifying energy between you and everything in your environment.

A GUIDED INTROVERSION TO TRY

On the Peloton app, the kind of meditations we offer are guided, meaning someone quietly talks you through the meditation, guiding your thought process according to a certain theme, whether it's a body scan for relaxation or inspiration to feel more forgiveness, courage, gratitude, or empathy. Guided meditations are excellent for beginners. Experienced meditators may prefer silent meditation with guidance—just sitting in contemplation, watching their thoughts, following the breath, or pondering a question.

Try this one, or any of the turning-in practices in the final chapter. In chapter 9, I'll give you a program for making introversion a habit, in which you can try different kinds of introversions as you gradually increase the time you spend in introversion. Here, however, I want to offer you a guided meditation to try, so you can begin to practice introversion in a more structured way.

Whether you've never really done what you consider to be "real meditation" or you're an experienced meditator, this and the other introversion practices in this book have a more traditional meditation flavor for you to dip your toe in. Any of these can be appropriate for daily use, or you can do them as needed. And again, for more meditations and a complete program that can help you ease into meditation and develop your own introversion practice, see chapter 9.

INTROVERSION TO START THE DAY FEELING GROUNDED AND FREE

Sometimes you want to relax, but at the start of the day, introversion can help you focus and get into the right mindset for what's to come. You can also use this meditation for a reset when you need to wipe the slate clean and feel ready to give yourself a fresh perspective. The theme of this morning meditation is to create a solid foundation for the day, from which you can expand in whatever direction you need today, for a sense of creativity and openness.

1. Sit comfortably, supported if necessary with a bolster, cushion, pillows, or blankets. Close your eyes. Breathe naturally for a few moments and feel the breath moving in and out of you.
2. Imagine moving your focus into the center of your brain. Imagine a tiny version of yourself in the space between your eyes.
3. Imagine walking down a flight of stairs from between your eyes to the top of your spinal column or the base of your brain.

4. Imagine a jewel representing your being and aliveness. See it in front of you, pulsing and glowing with life.

5. Imagine a gentle but powerful cascading waterfall that flows down from the top of your head, cleansing your energy as it goes and rinsing the jewel clean so it sparkles as it glows. This waterfall flows all the way down your spine, into your pelvis, where it pools, creating a calm lagoon space.

6. Now, imagine your avatar walking through a door at the base of your chest, down a hallway that leads into your heart.

7. Find yourself standing in the cavern of the heart, looking around at the warm golden energy of the heart. This cavern is alive with emotions, experiences, and hopes.

8. Like a movie camera that begins to pull away, widening the scope, widen and expand away from the core of your heart, in every direction simultaneously.

9. Imagine that you are embodying an ever-increasing, infinite expansion of space and freedom.

10. Very slowly, take a deep breath in through the mouth, then exhale through the mouth with a *haaaa* sound. Take another deep breath the same way.

11. Put your hands together in front of your chest, bow your head, and make a wish or a blessing for your day that you can take that feeling of safety and groundedness or openness and freedom into your day in whatever way you need.

12. Release your hands and slowly open your eyes.

T.I.P.

If your goal is to start introverting—maybe you want to call it meditating—on a regular basis, but you don't want to do a guided meditation, start easy. If your goals are too challenging, you probably won't keep it up. The best way to create a new habit is to start small. Maybe you do a structured sitting meditation once a month, or once a week. Maybe you will sit and breathe for three minutes every Wednesday at noon, or you will turn inward and contemplate how your inner body feels every time you brush your teeth. Setting a cadence that is both realistic and pushes the envelope just a little bit can help you to become habitual about meditation, if that's what you desire. Find a balance between what is realistic and idealistic.

Here is a basic daily meditation for you to try. You can expand the time you spend on this infinitely, but I suggest starting at three to five minutes, then working up from there. Or, if you want to work your way up in a more systemized manner, check out the next chapter, for a four-week program to establish a regular introversion practice.

Spend as much time as you like at each step.

1. Sit comfortably, supported if necessary. Close your eyes.
2. Draw your attention to your breath. Feel it moving in and out of you.
3. Let your breath bring your attention inside.
4. Begin to feel your breath from the inside out. How does your breath feel differently when you are turning inward?
5. Stay with your breath. Keep your focus on it. As thoughts come into your mind, which they will, watch them as if

you are outside of them. Watch them dance and play. See them with benevolent compassion, then bring your attention back to the breath.

6. Take a slow deep breath through your nose, then exhale slowly through your mouth, with a *haaaa* sound. Repeat three times.

7. Slowly open your eyes and reflect on your experience.

8. Do it again tomorrow.

CHAPTER 9

———

A FOUR-WEEK PLAN
TO ESTABLISH
AN INTROVERSION
PRACTICE

Throughout this book I've frequently extolled the virtues of a regular, systematic, intentional introversion practice. Here's where you can begin creating one, if you haven't already. This four-week plan starts you out at just five daily minutes of introversions you can insert into your day whenever you need them. That's week one.

In week two, you'll move up to ten daily minutes. Each day, you'll get a different technique to try, so you can begin to broaden your introversion repertoire. There are more traditional meditation techniques than the seven you'll find here, but I've included some of the more common types, so you can get familiar with them. Two primary types I don't include are guided meditations (when someone talks you through a meditation, which is essentially what I've been doing in all the meditations in this book) and visualizations, which you've also already tried many times in this book, whenever I have you imagine something. There are other types as well, but after you're done with this week, you'll be a little more familiar with breath counting, body scans, mantras, visual focusing, mindfulness, loving kindness, and walking meditation.

Week three moves you up to fifteen minutes per day. You can use the guided meditations I've provided here, or begin trying to go unguided, using any of the techniques you learned from week two, or elsewhere in this book.

Finally, in week four, you'll hit the sweet spot that is a twenty-minute daily meditation. This is enough time to go really deep, and I'll provide you with some more advanced guided meditations. Or, again, you can go it alone and see what happens when you sit for twenty minutes and plunge into the depths of your inner landscape.

Note that the timing of these meditations is solely for helping you to extend your practice. It's not strict. If you go longer than five minutes during the first week, or can only do two minutes, that's fine. In fact, during any meditation in these entire four weeks, you can always go longer, and on some days, you might need to cut it short for any number of reasons, internal or external. That's okay, too. Never forget that you can't do it wrong. This program just offers guidelines to assist you in building a practice; it's not intended to enforce strict rules upon you.

Also note that if you want to skip and try introversion less frequently at first, the next chapter has a list of meditations you can try at any time. You're more than welcome to start there if you don't have time now for a four-week practice.

MUSIC FOR MEDITATION?

People sometimes wonder if they should play music during meditation. If you do meditations on the Peloton app, you'll notice that they always include music in the background. I like to use music, but some people find it distracting. If it pulls your attention away from your practice, it may not be for you, or it may not be the right music. A quiet, relaxing, meditative music without anyone singing words or without an obvious melody line works best for most people. If you have meditation music you like, you can certainly feel free to use it with these introversion practices. You might also try it without music, to see how that changes your experience. The litmus test is: Does it help you to introvert, or does it pull you to extrovert?

For each meditation, especially during weeks two, three, and four, read the meditation first, then open your eyes to read each step, do that step, then move to the next step. Or, record yourself reading the instructions and play it back. The benefit of recording your instructions is that you can use that recording over and over whenever you want to do that meditation again.

I hope you'll love this experience, and if you like structure, you can follow it exactly as written. Or again, feel free to take liberties. You don't have to introvert, or meditate, every day if it doesn't fit into your schedule or you just feel like you need to go at a slower pace. You could start with every other day and work up to daily . . . or not. You could switch the meditations around, or swap them out with other meditations from the previous chapters that you enjoyed, or make up your own guided meditations—or just sit there, turn inward, and see what you find. It's your practice, not mine.

(And if you're looking for more, feel free to join me on the Peloton app and say hello! Use #turninginward or #introversion and I'll be sure to see you.)

WEEK ONE: FIVE MINUTES

During week one, we'll keep it nice and easy. You've already done (or at least read) many Quick T.I.P.s throughout these chapters, and that's the level we're going for this week. You could sit down in the morning, midday, or evening to do these five-minute introversions, or do them on the go. If you think you might forget, set a Quick T.I.P. reminder in your phone. Try to get one in every day.

When you're ready, read through the guidance, set a timer for five minutes (or make it approximate), then go through the guided introversion, either from memory or by reading each step and then practicing it. After, sit quietly for the remainder of the five minutes, contemplating your experience and noticing how you feel.

I've provided seven days of introversions here, but you could also substitute any of these Quick T.I.P.s with any of the other ones in this book you've already encountered and enjoyed.

DAY ONE: Wonder Moment

At any moment during the day today, take a moment to look at the world with wonder, as if through the eyes of a child. This is a poetic focus exercise that teaches your mind to concentrate, but that also bridges the binary of adulthood, which is a more extroverted state, and childhood, which is a more introverted, playful, mystical state that revels in the joy of unknowing. This is a nice introversion to do when you happen to be outside, although you can also do it inside, as long you can see something physically moving.

1. Wherever you are, scan your environment for something that is subtly moving in an interesting way. It could be the sun slowly setting, or raindrops sliding down a windowpane, a slight breeze through the leaves on a tree, or even a tissue in a box, moving very slightly in the air of a ceiling fan—anything random that catches your eye, big or small, obvious or barely noticeable.

2. Watch that thing. Wonder at it. Imagine you've never seen or noticed it before. Marvel at its dramatic or subtle beauty, its complexity, its mystery. Try to see it through the eyes of a child. Let it absorb all your attention, as if it is the most fascinating thing you've ever seen.

DAY TWO: Acts of Service

This exercise is good for when you are out in the world, but feeling anxious or stuck in your own head. It may not feel like an introversion because you are actively doing something, but it comes from a space of introversion, so it counts. (Note: While there are of course much larger ways to serve and help, sometimes a small act of service can turn your day, and someone else's day, around.)

1. Wherever you are, stop what you are doing and look around. Scan your environment.

2. Does anyone look like they need help? Is anyone noticeably struggling?

3. Some things you might find you could do: Open a door for someone, help someone pick up something they dropped, get something off a store shelf for someone who can't reach, let someone who seems to be in a hurry go ahead of you in line, offer to help someone find their way if they are lost, give someone who is homeless some spare change or a few dollars, even offer an understanding word to a harried parent dealing with a child having a tantrum or someone who looks like they are having a bad day. Give someone a compliment.

4. After you've done some small act of service, notice if you feel a shift in your mood or anxiety level.

DAY THREE: Superhero

A quick way to generate a feeling of virtuosic courage is to imagine yourself as a superhero! Have you ever noticed that after you see a superhero movie, when you come out of the theater, you have this feeling that you have powers? (Is it just me, ha-ha?) Because we have that capacity within, imagining we are superheroes can take us out of our normal, extroverted identifications of limited agency, into a sense of inner mystical belief in our own superpower.

1. When you are in a safe space where you won't feel self-conscious, imagine you have suddenly been granted superhero powers.

2. Puff up your chest and feel this power viscerally, as if you've been turned into Thor or Wonder Woman (or any other superhero you relate to).

3. Take the posture and stance that feels super-heroic to you. Feel the superhero energy coursing through you.

4. Tap into this feeling throughout the day. There really is a mystical power you have within you. The superhero image is just a way for you to begin feeling it.

DAY FOUR: Peaceful Moment

To break the momentum of tension, you can (ironically) create tension and then consciously release it, so a feeling of peace organically arises.

1. Take a moment in a place where you won't feel self-conscious tensing your muscles.

2. Sitting or standing comfortably, relax and take a few deep breaths.

3. Ball your hands into fists and squeeze them as hard as you can.

4. While continuing to squeeze your fists, pull your shoulders up and contract your shoulder and arm muscles.

5. Tighten your ab muscles and glute muscles, then your thighs and calf muscles.

6. Let your whole body feel fully tensed and contracted for a few more seconds.

7. Let go of all the contractions and let everything relax. Feel a sense of peace and relaxation flowing into your body.

8. Notice how you feel after doing this. Do you feel more inner peace and a release of tension? If not, you can repeat this several times.

DAY FIVE: *Kinesthetic Awareness*

For this meditation, you will associate physical states of stress and relaxation with mental feelings.

1. Go to a place where you can focus quietly for a few minutes. Sit or stand comfortably.
2. Make a fist, with one or both hands. Hold your fist as tightly as you can.
3. Name things you associate with tightness, such as stress, pain, anxiety, regret.
4. Release your fist and let your fingers relax.
5. Name things you associate with relaxation, such as calm, freedom, health, gentleness.
6. Repeat several times, physically feeling tension and associating it with words that come to mind, then physically feeling relaxation and associating it with words that come to mind.

DAY SIX: *Relaxation Intervention*

This is a good introversion for a moment when you feel a lot of stress or tension.

1. Sit or lie down comfortably, supported if necessary, so you feel completely physically relaxed and no part of your body has to hold tension or support you uncomfortably.
2. Take a few deep breaths, slowly extending your exhalation so it is longer than your inhalation.

3. Imagine that you are slowly rising from where you are sitting or lying down. You feel entirely safe, with a magical capacity to rise literally above your world.

4. Look down at the world as you slowly float higher and higher. As everything below you grows smaller, notice how insignificant it all looks from above.

5. Let yourself feel a detachment set in: you can see your life below, but you aren't connected to it in this moment.

6. Let your face and back soften and relax as you continue to rise, observe, and feel freer and freer from the constraints and stresses of that busy world below.

7. Now, imagine you are floating back down, slowly, slowly, back into your body, but let the feeling of calm detachment persist. You've put things in perspective.

8. Open your eyes and notice if you feel differently.

DAY SEVEN: Finding Gratitude

We all know gratitude is a good thing, but sometimes it can be hard to generate. In this introversion, you'll discover a gratitude that you don't have to manufacture because it's already inside of you.

1. Sit comfortably, supported if necessary. Close your eyes.

2. Bring your attention inside of you, right into the middle of your chest, and further, all the way inside your heart.

3. Imagine that inside your heart is a chamber and you are standing inside that chamber. The chamber is lit as if by candlelight, and the walls softly pulse with the slow beating of your heart.

4. Imagine that within this chamber, you notice the sudden formation of a source of light, right in the middle of the chamber, hovering just at the level of your eyes. The light glows and pulses with your heartbeat, and begins to grow, softly illuminating the chamber.

5. You know the light is a gift to you. It is the gift of your own life, of your beating heart, of your mind that is able to visualize all of this, of *you*, in all your depth and beauty.

6. Reach out to the light and pull it into yourself. Feel the spreading gratitude of being given this gift of life, light, and love.

7. Fold your hands in front of your heart in a prayer position and let this sweet, almost overwhelming gratitude fill you as you offer profound thanks for the gift you've been given: the gift of yourself.

8. Slowly lower your hands, open your eyes, and notice how you feel.

9. Bonus introversion: Notice if your day goes any differently after this meditation.

WEEK TWO: TEN MINUTES

This week, we're upping the stakes. You're going to be doing a ten-minute introversion practice each day. Ten minutes isn't a long time, but it's double what you were doing before, so get ready to go deeper.

This week's introversions are a little more structured, so it may be easier to do them at a set time, such as in the morning or evening, rather than doing them during the day or while you're doing other things. These introversions each use more traditional techniques, although I often put my own spin on them to make them a bit more accessible. As you try these, notice how they make you feel. You are likely to have some favorites, and there may be some that don't appeal to you as much. This will be important information for the future of your practice.

As with week one, read the meditation first, then set a timer, but this time for ten minutes. Remember or reread the instructions, and when you've finished, continue to contemplate or repeat the practice until the ten minutes have passed.

DAY ONE: Counting the Breath

This is one of the most basic forms of meditation. The purpose of counting your breaths is to focus on something, to train your mind to maintain that one-pointed focus. This is the same goal of many other types of traditional meditations that you'll try this week, including using a mantra or focusing on a visual point. Some people love to do this kind of meditation because it's so simple. Other people think it's boring. Give it a try and see how it works for you.

You may be surprised to find that you can't get to a count of ten without your mind wandering and that is totally okay. The mind wanders. Remember the puppies on the playground. When you notice that the puppies (your thoughts) have distracted you, no judgment. No hurry. Just go back to your count, wherever you left off, or start back at one. It's tempting to make this a goal-oriented exercise, but I find it's more effective if it's not. You're giving your mind an internal activity, and sometimes it takes a break. And that's okay.

That being said, you may find that the more often you do this, the more easily you will stay focused and reach ten, and even back to one, without getting too distracted. When you reach this stage, you may also notice that you become better at concentrating or focusing on things in your daily life.

1. Sit or lie down in a comfortable position, supported if necessary. Set a timer for ten minutes.
2. Close your eyes and bring your attention to your breath. Feel it moving in and out of you but don't try to control it.
3. Now, begin counting your breaths. Inhale, count (in your mind, say *one*), then exhale.
4. Repeat until you get to ten breaths, thinking the number of your count at the top of the inhale.
5. When you get to ten, count backward, back down to one.
6. Whenever your mind wanders (and it will), as soon as you notice, just go back to your counting.
7. Continue until your ten minutes is up, then take a moment to notice how you feel.

DAY TWO: *Body Scan*

This is another common type of meditation that I really love, especially for beginners and also for experienced meditators. It helps get back to the basics of turning inward. The body scan doesn't try to still or focus the thoughts. Instead, this technique anchors the thoughts into different parts of the body. This can help you to focus more organically because your thoughts aren't still. They're moving, but it's you moving them on purpose.

As you engage in this introversion, I'd like you to do so with a feeling of openness and acceptance of who you are. As you move gently through each part of your body, focusing your attention on that part, try to do so with a tender compassion and love for your own body, which works so hard and does so much to carry you through this life. As you move through this introversion, go slowly and really focus your attention on each part.

1. Sit or lie down comfortably, supported if necessary. Set a timer for ten minutes.
2. Close your eyes and take a few deep breaths.
3. Bring your attention to the top of your head. Feel it (without touching it), then imagine it softening and relaxing, almost as if it's melting down over your scalp.
4. Let that warm melting feeling run down over your ears. Bring your attention to your ears as they soften and relax, then over the hinge of your jaw.
5. Shift your attention to the back and sides of your neck, as the warm melting feeling relaxes your entire head and face.

6. Now bring your attention into your upper back and shoulders as they soften and relax.

7. The melting feeling is moving down the sides of your ribs and over your belly. Bring your attention to your torso and feel it relaxing.

8. Shift your attention to your hips as all the tension flows out of them. Let your attention move along with the melting feeling, spreading down your thighs and into your knees, down your calves and feet, all the way to the tips of your toes.

9. Slowly take a deep breath in, then fully exhale. Stay here for a few more minutes, feeling how relaxed your entire body is. If you feel any tension creeping back in anywhere, send your attention to that place.

10. If you still have time, let your attention move to different parts of your body and affix it there, always infusing the area you're focusing on with that warm melting feeling.

11. When your time is done, float your hands into a prayer position in front of your heart. Bow your head and recognize if you feel differently or have discovered something useful. Imprint it and wish it forward into your day.

12. Release your hands and gently open your eyes.

DAY THREE: Using a Mantra

A mantra is essentially a word or phrase that is repeated or chanted as a point of focus during meditation. Mantra meditation is one of the more traditional forms of meditation, and it's both easy and challenging. There is a stereotype of meditation in which someone sits cross-legged on the floor and chants the word "*om*" (an approximate translation of this Sanskrit word is "message"). *Om* is thought to be a mystical word that imitates the primordial pulsation or the sound of the creation of all things, and some people like the way it vibrates within when they chant it. However, a mantra can be anything—a sacred word or a commonplace word.

In some forms of meditation, such as transcendental meditation (TM), a teacher initiates the student into a certain meditation technique and gives the student a private mantra. More often, people who use mantra meditation choose a word like *om*, or a word with some meaning to them, such as *grace, joy, peace, calm, clarity,* or *love,* or a phrase or affirmation, such as *I am love, I find peace within, I am strong.* In the yoga tradition, it's common to use a Sanskrit mantra that references one of the Hindu gods or goddesses, such as *namah shivaya,* or *ham sa, so hum,* as I mentioned in the context of moving meditation on page 173.

What mantra should you use? Any mantra you like. Choose from anything I've mentioned here, or use another word that has meaning and resonance for you, and follow these very simple steps. With practice, just as with counting the breath, you may begin to notice that you have an easier time concentrating and focusing in your daily life.

1. Think about a word or phrase you would like to use as a mantra.
2. Sit comfortably, back straight, supported if necessary. Set a timer for ten minutes.
3. Try to feel a lightness to your spine, as if it is rising up rather than sinking down.
4. Take a few deep breaths, close your eyes, then either silently or out loud, say your mantra.

5. Repeat the mantra, either in rhythm with your breath, or randomly and specifically not in rhythm with your breath (see the box below about which to try and why).

6. If your mind wanders, you are not doing it wrong. This is natural. As soon as you notice, just bring your attention back gently to the mantra.

7. Repeat until your timer goes off, then open your eyes and notice how you feel.

MANTRAS AND RHYTHMIC ATTUNEMENT

One of the benefits of working with a mantra while meditating is the rhythm of the chant, which may be more important than the mantra itself because it brings the body into a state of rhythm and resonance.

People often wonder whether they should say the mantra in their minds in rhythm or out loud, and they also wonder whether they should say (or think) the mantra in rhythm with their breath (or in the case of walking meditation, in rhythm with their step—see page 173). Or, is it better to say the mantra in a rhythm that is not related to anything external?

There are differing opinions on this. Some people think you should say a mantra out loud because of the vibration that can physically happen in your body from making the sound. Others say it doesn't matter. As for whether you should say the mantra in rhythm, I believe there are pros and cons to synching up a mantra with what you are doing in your body.

An upside to rhythmic attunement is that it can be a therapy for people who have some kind of asynchronous health issue. For people with multiple sclerosis or another autoimmune disease or degenerative illness, rhythmically attuning the mantra to the step or the breath can bring harmony to the body. One of the theories (although there have been no studies on this that I know of) is that when the body is fighting itself, as it does with an autoimmune disease, it is in a state of asynchrony. Heart conditions can also be based in asynchrony, such as with irregular heart rhythms like atrial fibrillation. Walking and breathing and creating patterns and rhythms might help—again, no evidence, but there's the hope/theory that this could be helpful for those conditions.

The downside to chanting in the rhythm of your breath (or step) is that you risk the mantra becoming rote. When your mantra is on automatic pilot in the background, it's no longer directing your attention internally. It's no longer focusing you or balancing you. When a mantra that used to take you into a flow state becomes routine, it can actually cause you to extrovert rather than introvert, as if the mantra is getting in the way—an annoying noise in the background. Or, you can become dependent on it, unable to introvert without it. Or, it can simply lose its juice so it's not doing anything for you anymore. You can become more concerned with the absence of the flow state than you are with allowing the flow state to happen.

That's when it's time to shake things up a little bit and not do the mantra in time with your step, or even do it asynchronously.

DAY FOUR: *Visual Focusing*

In this type of meditation, you use a visual point rather than a word or sound to focus on. A common practice is to focus on a candle flame, but you could focus on anything—an object such as a photo or a figurine, the center of a mandala (an intricate circular image that is basically a kind of spiritual art used for the purpose of meditation), or anything else that feels inspiring to you. Traditionally, as you focus visually on this object, you go for as long as you can without blinking, only looking away when you need to blink and closing your eyes for a few seconds. However, this practice is in my opinion just as effective and potentially less uncomfortable if you blink as necessary. As with other practices that use a point of focus, you may notice after doing this regularly that you are better able to focus and concentrate in your daily life.

1. Choose the object you will focus on, such as a candle flame. (Be safe with a lighted candle!) Set a timer for ten minutes.
2. Sit comfortably, supported if necessary, with the object in front of you. Rest your hands in your lap or on your knees with palms down or up. Take a few deep breaths.
3. Focus on the object with a soft, relaxed gaze. Notice everything about it. Keep your focus on that actual object in front of you, blinking normally as you feel the need.
4. If your mind wanders and you stop noticing what you're looking at, that's fine and in fact likely. When you notice, softly redirect your focus back to the object.

5. If your eyes get tired, close them for a moment. If you see an imprint of the object when you close your eyes (such as the candle flame), focus on that. When your eyes feel ready, open them again and resume your focus.

6. Continue looking at the object until the timer goes off.

7. Take another deep breath, blink a few times, and notice if there is any change in how you feel.

DAY FIVE: Mindfulness

I've talked about mindfulness in the section on presence of mind on page 68, but as an introversion practice, mindfulness has the interesting quality of focusing on what is external in order to turn inward. It is the thread of extroversion in your introversion. In this meditation, your point of focus is...everything. That is, everything in the present moment. It's about noticing exactly where you are and how it feels, inside and out.

You can choose your surroundings, your sensory impressions (like the exercise on page 73), or how you feel inside as a point of focus. Or all of these, as you shift back and forth in order to experience all aspects of the now, which is what I'll have you do in the instructions. This is the beginner level. As you get better at focusing on what's happening right now, you can spend more time with a more diffuse experience of simply being present without putting your focus on any one thing. (Or, you could try jumping right to this process right now, simply setting a timer for ten minutes and just being there, redirecting your attention when it goes into the past or future without following the cues below.) Doing this regularly can help you to be more present in your daily life.

Some people find mindfulness practices to be less effortful than practices that focus on just one thing. Because you keep shifting your focus to different aspects of your environment, it can be easier, especially at first, to stay with your focus. That being said, remember that your mind will wander and that is all part of the process, not anything you're doing wrong.

1. Sit comfortably, supported if necessary. Set a timer for ten minutes. Take a few deep breaths.

2. From where you are sitting, without turning your head, softly notice everything you can see around you. Put a label on what you notice. Try to see neutrally, without adding any judgment or opinion. Not "this room is messy" but instead, "couch," "table," "pillow," "ceiling fan," etc.

3. As you continue to look, also notice what you hear, and give it a label: "traffic noise," "birds singing," "wind," "furnace fan," "someone talking."

4. Now, take everything in generally. Be present in the room, continuing to notice what's happening right now.

5. When your mind starts to wander to something else, like something that happened in the past or something you're going to do, or need to do, in the future, that's okay. Remind yourself that your thoughts are like puppies on the playground. When you notice you're doing this, gently bring your attention back to an awareness of the present moment.

6. Now, run through all your senses, just a moment for each one: notice what you see right now, what you hear right now, what you smell right now, what you taste

right now, what is touching you right now. Go through these as if you are browsing through channels on a radio.

7. Next, turn inward and notice everything you feel in your body. Go through the different parts, almost like a mini body scan: How does your head feel? Your neck and shoulders? Your stomach? How do your arms feel? Your hands? Your legs and feet? Notice where you might be feeling good, or feeling pain, or feeling tension.

8. Now, put them all together, scanning through the external environment, your senses, your internal environment.

9. For the last few minutes of this meditation, stop scanning your environment and see if you can diffusely focus on the present moment without a particular point of focus. Just feel yourself being right here, right now. Stay here until the timer goes off.

10. Take a deep breath, and notice how you feel.

DAY SIX: Loving Kindness

An introversion focusing on loving kindness is based on a type of meditation called *Metta*, which is the Pali word (a language from northern India) that can be loosely translated as "kindness to others." This is my version of that concept, in which you send positive energy to other people in your life. We all have different reactions to the idea of, or the word, "kindness." If you have a difficult relationship with that word, that's okay. If that's you, you can change the focus to another word that feels positive to you, such as compassion, patience, or even detachment. The Sanskrit word for the emotional source of kindness is *bhava*. This meditation is incredibly healing if you are having trouble communicating with or getting along with someone, and also in general, as sending love outward generates more inner compassion.

1. Sit or lie down comfortably, supported if necessary. Set a timer for ten minutes.
2. Close your eyes and take a few deep breaths.
3. Think of someone you love, either now or in the past, either a personal relationship or a guide or teacher. Imagine that person is sitting in front of you. Imagine you can hear them breathing, as you can hear yourself breathing.
4. Imagine your heart filling with love, kindness, or whatever word you are using for this meditation. Imagine offering this love and kindness to that person, projecting it forward. Imagine them taking that love and kindness into their heart.
5. Spend a few minutes basking in the feeling of this offering and their acceptance of it.
6. Now, think of someone who pushes your buttons, rubs you the wrong way, or with whom you have any kind of difficult relationship. Maybe you don't want them in your life, or maybe you can't do anything about the fact that they are in your life. Maybe they aren't in your life anymore, but you still carry some anger or animosity towards them.
7. Imagine that person is sitting in front of you. You can hear them breathing, just as you can hear yourself breathing.

8. To the best of your ability, generate a feeling of kind-ness, love, patience, compassion, or detachment towards them. Offer that person this energy. Imagine them taking it into their own heart. If this is really difficult, know that this doesn't mean you have to start liking the person or accepting their behavior, or even forgiving them in this moment. This is purely a healing measure for you and for the relationship, even if it has ended or will end.

9. Spend a few minutes feeling the energy of this offering.

10. Now, this last part is difficult for some people. Be coura-geous and think of the parts of you that you have trou-ble accepting. Step back and see yourself as someone who needs love and deserves compassion.

11. Imagine an image of you sitting across from you. Hear your breathing, both there and within you. Feel love and kindness for yourself rising within your heart. Offer it to yourself, and imagine yourself accepting the offering with gratitude and love.

12. Stay here, basking in the *bhava* you've accessed. Envision it as a luminous energy expanding beyond your body, radiating out from you.

13. When the timer goes off, take a deep breath. Fold your hands in a prayer position in front of your heart and bow your head in reverence to the power of loving kindness.

14. Lower your hands in your lap, raise your head, and very slowly open your eyes. Notice if you feel any different towards others and also towards yourself.

DAY SEVEN: *Walking Meditation*

I gave you one version of a walking meditation on page 173, but this version doesn't include a mantra. It's similar to a mindfulness meditation but while you are on the move. In a traditional *kinhin* walking meditation, meditators walk in a slow circle together and can focus more internally, but when you are walking around in the world, such as in a natural area, this version of walking meditation keeps your focus on what's going on around you, which is of course a safer way to meditate while moving. Many people find that they can introvert best and reap the most benefits when they do it while moving rather than sitting or lying still. Even if you have a regular sitting practice, you might want to incorporate walking meditations, too.

Note that this is a ten-minute meditation, but it can be such a joyful experience that you may want to extend it. Of course you can continue longer (as you can with any practice in this chapter).

1. Choose somewhere you can walk that has a pleasant atmosphere and isn't too loud or distracting. Walking through a park, a forest, on a quiet beach, or anywhere you feel comfortable and calm works, although you can technically do this anywhere, even down a busy city street. Set a timer you carry with you (such as on your phone or watch) for ten minutes. Take a few deep breaths.
2. Begin walking at a slow pace in a regular rhythm. Take each step with care and intention.
3. Bring your attention to your breath, noticing the rhythm of the inhale and exhale. Imagine that when you inhale, your energy rises through your body, and as you exhale,

the energy moves downward, relaxing and softening your skin.

4. Synch your steps with your breath, such as four steps as you inhale, four steps as you exhale, counting the steps in your mind: inhale and step 1-2-3-4, exhale and step 1-2-3-4.

5. Once you are comfortable with walking and breathing in a synchronized way, slow your inhale and exhale, without slowing your steps. If you were using a count of four, expand that to a count of five, so that you take five steps to inhale and five steps to exhale.

6. Slow your inhale and exhale again, to a count of six: inhale and step 1-2-3-4-5-6, exhale and step 1-2-3-4-5-6.

7. Once you get comfortable walking and breathing at this pace, let your awareness expand to your surroundings. Notice everything you see, hear, smell, and feel around you.

8. Imagine your energy expanding into your surroundings as you walk. Bask in the beauty, even of the ordinary things. Marvel at the creation of the material world. Stay here until the timer goes off.

9. Take a few deep breaths as you head back to where you started, and begin to walk and breathe normally. Continue noticing your environment and as you walk, contemplate whether you feel any different than you did before you started.

WEEK THREE: FIFTEEN MINUTES

This week's introversions are even more structured, as you expand your introversion time to fifteen minutes. They are a little longer and a little more complex and will give you even more ideas for techniques and ways to guide your attention within. That being said, you can also use any of the meditations from week two (or elsewhere in this book) and just extend the time in them to fifteen minutes. By the way, note that since this meditation is longer, it's possible you will get some discomfort. If you feel uncomfortable, it's completely fine to move, stretch your legs, change position, lie down, or take a break. My hope is that knowing you can remain comfortable will keep you engaged in the introversion longer.

DAY ONE: Peace Be with You

This introversion focuses on generating or accessing a sense of inner peace. It's good for days when you're feeling anxious or agitated, but it can also be a lovely way to start or end your day. You have an inner peace that is already there but may be cloaked by stresses and the natural pressures of life. In this meditation, you'll be working on unveiling that peace that already exists within you.

1. Sit or lie down comfortably, supported if necessary. Rest your hands in your lap or with your palms down on your knees. Set a timer for fifteen minutes.
2. Close your eyes and take a few deep breaths. Notice if you are feeling any negative or resistant feelings right at the beginning, even if it's just that you don't really feel

like sitting here. That is human and okay. This is why you're here—to engage with and reorient that feeling.

3. Feel the floor below you and visualize the earth beneath the foundation of where you are sitting.

4. Begin to imagine roots growing down from your legs and pelvis, as if you were a tree. These roots are anchoring you to the earth beneath you.

5. Envision that your torso is the trunk of this tree. Feel the front, sides, and back of your torso and imagine this as the literal trunk of a tree. This tree is formidable, ancient, courageous, persistent. See if you can sense the power and fortitude of a great tree manifesting in the form of you.

6. Imagine the branches and leaves of the tree that is an expression of you, surrounding you and extending all around you in all directions. Feel the grandeur of this tree—its magnificence and reach.

7. Now you will imagine five different kinds of winds passing through the leaves of the tree. Even though the branches and leaves will move, the trunk and roots—the deep inner peace underlying the winds of stress—remain unmoved, stolid, and strong.

8. The first wind is the pressure to feel safe. This is a wind symbolizing our deepest survival needs. Imagine this wind blowing through the branches. Feel the solid core of peace in the trunk of your tree, as you let the wind blow through the branches and away.

9. The second wind is the pressure of expectations based on the stories we tell about ourselves, or that people tell us about ourselves. What are we expected to be and do?

The wind passes through the branches and you can feel it moving and thrashing, but within the trunk and roots, there remains a solid core of peace.

10. The third wind is the pressure of relationships. Any relationships, positive, neutral, negative, their energy blows through the branches and leaves, but within the trunk and roots, there remains a solid core of peace.

11. The fourth wind is the pressure of growth. Feel the pressure of wanting to do better, to expand and evolve, racing through the branches like a whirlwind, then moving away, as the trunk and roots remain a solid core of peace.

12. The fifth wind is the pressure of the desire to be free. The wind blows through, wild and frenetic, but within the trunk and roots, there remains a solid core of peace.

13. Take a deep breath in. Let the visual images fade, and bathe in the light of your own experience with this meditation. Stay here until the timer goes off.

14. Slowly fold your hands in front of your heart and bow your head. Take a moment to honor any seeds of peace you've planted. Wish it forward into the rest of your day.

15. Release your hands and gently open your eyes. Feel any difference in your body and mind.

DAY TWO: *Foot Breathing and Spine Steeling*

This meditation uses the image of breathing through your feet and creating stability in the spine. You can do this one sitting in a chair or standing, as long as the soles of your feet can be placed on the ground. However, start in a chair if you think it will be difficult in any way to stay standing in one position for fifteen minutes.

This meditation is useful for feeling more grounded when you are having trouble focusing on what you need to do. It's also good for any time you want to feel like you've metaphorically got your feet on the ground.

1. Sit in a chair or stand comfortably, supported if necessary. Remove shoes and socks, and place your bare feet on the ground (inside or outside). If you are standing, don't lock your knees. Set a timer for fifteen minutes.

2. Take a long, slow, deep breath in. Exhale through your mouth, long and slow. Take another deep breath in. Exhale through your nose this time. Close your eyes.

3. Bring your attention to your feet. Notice how they feel against the floor or ground.

4. Begin to bring a feeling of heaviness to your feet. Let this heaviness extend up into your hips, so that your entire body, from hips to feet, has a heavy, immovable quality.

5. Take a deep breath in again, but this time, imagine exhaling through your feet. Feel the breath pouring out of the soles of your feet. Breathe in again, then out through your feet. One more time, in, and out through your feet.

6. In your mind, trace your spine from your pelvis, all the way to the crown of your head. Imagine imbuing your spine with titanium-like strength. Feel how nothing is more powerful than your core. Spend a few minutes adjusting to these new feelings in your body: heavy feet, heavy hips, adamantine core.

7. Feeling that unwavering fortitude in your core, soften the muscles in your face, relax your shoulders away from your ears, and imagine that the surface of your body is safe in

relaxation because of your internal strength. Spend a few minutes noticing the difference between the strength of your foundation and core and the softness of your muscles and skin.

8. Return to the feeling of inhaling and then exhaling through the soles of your feet, as you feel them heavy on the floor or ground. See if you can feel it all at once: the foot breathing, the spine steeling, the heavy base and the soft exterior of your body. Stay here in contemplation of the many energies coordinating within you, until the timer goes off.

9. Take a deep breath and open your eyes. Tune in to your energy. Do you feel a shift? Notice how and in what ways.

DAY TWO: *Listening and Listing, Part 1*

This two-part meditation begins by helping you to focus deeply on just one of your five senses by singling out all the things you can hear. In some ways, listening is an extroversion because you are directing your attention outward towards sounds you can hear, but in this case, this is more of an absence of attention to anything other than sound, so it becomes more of an introversion.

1. Sit or lie down comfortably, supported if necessary. Set a timer for fifteen minutes.

2. Close your eyes and take a few deep breaths.

3. Slowly tune in to all the sounds you can hear. In a quiet place, the sounds may be subtle. At first you may only hear the loudest sounds. As you hear each thing, name it,

such as: music, rustling papers, a car horn, people talking in the next room.

4. Now see if you can notice more subtle sounds: birds, whispering, the mechanical breath of an air conditioner or furnace, the sound of far-away traffic or a train, the hum of the refrigerator.

5. See if you can hear even more subtle sounds: you or someone else breathing, your heartbeat, a light breeze, the distant sounds of vibration or rumbling you may not be able to identify. Even if you can't name them, hang a mental lantern on them so you note in some way that you have heard each sound separately.

6. Now, move into a more passive listening. Focus on sound only, but don't name what you hear. Just listen. Do the sounds change? In volume, in tone, in vibration? Move your attention along with the waves of sound coming in.

7. When your mind wanders into thoughts, notice benevolently, then go back to listening. Stay here until the timer goes off.

8. Take a deep breath and open your eyes. Notice if you feel more attuned to your environment, or feel different in any other way.

DAY THREE: Listening and Listing, Part 2

This second part of the meditation helps you to organize your thoughts in a conscious way, rather than letting them exist in a miasma of noise and chaos. This can be a helpful exercise if chaotic thoughts are keeping you awake at night. Sometimes, simply organizing them into a list, such as "things I have to do tomorrow," can help your mind to relax so you can fall asleep. Or, if what is distracting you is making sense of ambivalent emotions, your list could help you to organize the spectrum of your feelings.

This practice doesn't feel as much like an introversion as some of the others, especially when it's externally focused on what can seem like the minutiae of daily life, but it's effective at putting your mind at ease, and that is what can facilitate introversion.

1. Sit or lie down comfortably. Set a timer for fifteen minutes.
2. Close your eyes and take a few deep breaths.
3. Choose any area of your life that you want to have more organized or put into a list. It could be work-related, a list of things you need to do around your house, goals for the next week or month or year, a list of aspirations, or anything else weighing on your mind because you haven't organized it.
4. Begin to parcel out your agenda, list your goals, or articulate your to-do list. See if there are high-level categories for your list, or just a title expressing what the list is about.
5. Now, begin filling in the list. What do you want on the list? What do you think of but realize doesn't belong on that list? This could be something as simple as listing all the things you have to do today, as complex as the steps you have to take in order to achieve something difficult, or as personal as listing all the emotions and sensations you are feeling in this moment.
6. Continue to add to, contemplate, and revise your list until the timer goes off.

7. Take a deep breath, imagine folding up the list and putting it into an envelope, then putting the envelope in your pocket, or in a special place like a safe or a chest.

8. Slowly open your eyes. See if your mind feels less chaotic, or if you notice anything else.

DAY FOUR: Labeling

Labeling gives you an opportunity to categorize what you are thinking and feeling in the moment. This is a little like listing, but more about putting different things you notice into groups. This is introversion by way of a conscious awareness of what your mind is doing. It's a good way to put intense or troubling thoughts and feelings at arm's length, helping you to detach from them emotionally so you don't feel quite so controlled by them.

1. Sit or lie down comfortably, supported if necessary. Set a timer for fifteen minutes.

2. Close your eyes and take a few deep breaths.

3. Imagine a long line of boxes, or files in a file cabinet in front of you. None of the boxes or files have anything written on them yet.

4. Now, begin to notice the thoughts in your head and the feelings that arise. You don't need to try to generate any thoughts or feelings. Just notice what comes up naturally.

5. Pick one of the thoughts or feelings, and give it a category. Imagine that one of the boxes or folders has this category written on it. If you think about how you'll be getting a haircut later that day, you could put that in the category "Things I am doing." If you think about what

you have to do this evening, you could put it in the category of "Schedule," or in the category of "Things I'm
looking forward to." If you think about a financial issue,
you could put it in the category of "Money" or in the category "Things I'm worrying about." If you notice a feeling of anxiety or worry, you could put it in the category
of "Anxieties" or "Worries," or "Feelings I don't like," or
just "Feelings." The categories can be called anything
that makes sense to you.

6. Imagine putting that thought or feeling in the box or
   folder with that category written on it.

7. Now, find another thought or feeling you happen to be
   having. Just turn in and look for it. When you find one,
   give it a category. Imagine another box or folder with that
   category written on it, and imagine putting the thought
   into that box or folder.

8. Thoughts and feelings will constantly flow into your
   mind, so continue to label them and put them in the
   appropriately labelled box or folder. Many may be in the
   same category, or each one might be in a different category. However you organize them is completely fine.
   There can be as many boxes, folders, and categories as
   you can think of. Just keep sticking each thought that
   arises naturally into its appropriate box or category.

9. After you've done this for a while, notice whether the
   thoughts and feelings that come up feel less personal and
   more like something you are witnessing neutrally rather
   than engaging with. Your only job is to put the thoughts
   into the right categories, not to let them carry you away.

10. If you get distracted, that's always fine. When you notice, just start back up with your filing system. If a thought or feeling persists, try to break it down into subcategories, putting each part into a box or folder.

11. Keep categorizing your thoughts and feelings as they arise until the timer goes off.

12. Take a deep breath and open your eyes. Notice if you feel more neutral or calmer, less confused, or anything else.

DAY FIVE: Compassion Consciousness

This meditation can help you to feel more compassion, empathy, or kindness towards someone else. Choose a particular person who you think is either in real need of compassion right now, or someone you're having trouble with right now, that you want to feel more compassion for but are struggling with that. This is a variation on the loving kindness meditation from week two, but with a focus on just one person.

1. Sit comfortably with any support you need. Set a timer for fifteen minutes.

2. Close your eyes and take a few deep breaths.

3. Think of someone you believe needs some kindness or compassion right now. This could be someone you know, or someone you know of.

4. Visualize that person sitting across from you, facing you. Spend some time simply observing the person—how they look, how they sit, how they look at you. Imagine you can hear them breathing.

5. Notice what feelings come up as you imagine looking at that person. What are your initial feelings? Do these feelings change as you look at them? Do they become more positive, or less positive? Do you naturally begin to feel some compassion or empathy, or do you start to feel some irritation, agitation, or sadness? Are your feelings more neutral, like curiosity or disinterest?

6. Now, imagine what that person sitting across from you might be feeling when they look at you. Are they feeling acceptance? Are they nervous? Are they sad, or hopeful? Angry, irritated, curious, optimistic? Are they seeking connection, or drawing away emotionally? Just imagine what they might be feeling, even if it wouldn't be accurate in real life.

7. Next, imagine that you can take your consciousness into your hands. It looks like a bright ball of light. Hand the ball of light to the person in front of you. Imagine they take that ball of light and press it into their own heart.

8. Feel what it's like for your consciousness to be inside that other person. What do you feel that they feel? Let yourself imagine how it feels to be inside that other person's heart.

9. Now, imagine the person slowly lifts the ball of light from their heart and hands it back to you. Return your consciousness to your own heart and contemplate the experience of feeling someone else's feelings.

10. Pass the ball of light back and forth, taking as much time as you need to experience what it feels like for your consciousness to be within someone else's heart, and what it

feels like to return your consciousness to your own heart. Notice how the energy between you and the imagined other person shifts as you continue to do this.

11. Keep engaging with the ball of light until the timer goes off. Then, gently place your hands on your heart as you imagine bringing your consciousness back into yourself.

12. Take a few deep breaths and bring your palms together in front of your heart. Bow to that other person, then slowly let their image fade away.

13. Lower your hands and slowly open your eyes. Notice if you feel differently about that person now. How have your feelings changed?

DAY SIX: Joy Consciousness

In this joyful introversion, you will cultivate a feeling of happiness. Joy feels different for each person, so let your own sense of what brings you joy spread internally in this meditation. You don't need any agenda other than uncloaking joy in your heart, in your own way. This isn't the easiest of introversions, but I would like to consider as you go through this that effort can be a catalyst for happiness. I also want to note that if you are in a difficult place and "joy" doesn't seem appropriate for you right now, you can translate the word "joy" to something like "courage" or "peace."

1. Sit or lie down comfortably, supported if necessary. Set a timer for fifteen minutes.

2. Close your eyes and take a few deep breaths.

3. Think about the word "joy." What does that word mean for you? If joy is what you are going for, keep that word.

If you want to use another word, you might choose happiness or gratitude or hope or something else.

4.   Now, search your memory or make up a story in which
     you were given a gift that made you feel organic,
     unplanned joy. It could be something a person gave
     you, or something you encounter in the world, like an
     unexpected, beautiful sunset. Feel that feeling of unex-
     pected joy.

5.   *Bhava* is the essence of an emotion—it's a somewhat eso-
     teric term that can also refer specifically to the internal
     source of kindness and joy. Turn inside and look for the
     source of the joy. This isn't about the gift itself, but about
     the feeling it engendered within you. Stay here feeling
     that feeling for a few moments.

6.   Now, look back in your memory, or make up a scenario,
     where you give a gift to someone else and witness an
     unplanned, organic joy arising from that person. You
     don't even have to know what the gift is. Just imagine
     that person opening the box, looking in, and how their
     face lights up as they feel joy.

7.   See if you can find the *bhava* in that other person—the
     deep source of their joy. Can you feel it in yourself as you
     witness it in them?

8.   Think about how the word "forgiveness" contains the
     word "give." If appropriate for you in this moment, see if
     you can remember something, or create a story, in which
     you give someone a gift, and that gift is forgiveness. Sit
     with this for a few moments to find a way to do this that
     feels okay, if you can. If not, remember the other word

you decided to use: Can you give someone the gift of patience, or courage, or peace?

9. Feel, if you can, how giving someone else this gift has an effect on you. Do you feel relief? Do you feel resistant, in which case you can hold back? Do you feel your own joy rising?

10. Take a huge breath, then a long exhale. Spend some time contemplating and feeling the source of joy within yourself.

11. Now, imagine the *bhava* rises above you, like a sun shining warmth and light on your face. Let yourself bathe within this joy-infused light, until the timer goes off.

12. Take another deep breath and slowly, sweetly fold your hands in front of your heart. Bow your head and honor your experience of this introversion.

13. Slowly lower your hands, lift your chin, and gently open your eyes.

14. Notice if you feel different, and in what ways.

DAY SEVEN: Embodying the Witness

The concept of this introversion is to step apart from thoughts and feelings in a neutral and detached way, for less stress and a sense of relief. This is a traditional meditation strategy, in which you become the witness to your thoughts and feelings, rather than the one actively experiencing your thoughts and feelings. This can have an incredible impact on how your day goes. Detachment is powerful, but to do this, you may need to take a leap of faith that this works. For most people, this is not a familiar way to think, but I urge you to try this.

It's a formidable tool for introversion. In this introversion, I'm going to walk you through multiple ways to embody the witness. You may resonate with some of these more than others. Whichever works for you, you can stick with that.

1. Sit or lie down comfortably, supported if necessary. Set a timer for fifteen minutes.
2. Close your eyes and take a few deep breaths.
3. Now, begin to feel and listen to your breath.
4. When you feel comfortable, imagine stepping apart from the breath and witnessing it with wonder. How amazing that you have this animating force moving in and out of you. Watch it as if you've never seen anyone breathing before. Stay here for a few minutes.
5. Now, imagine you are sitting in a beautiful old cinema. Nobody else is there. You have it all to yourself.
6. Imagine yourself in the front row. Look at the screen. On the screen, you see the thoughts and feelings you're having projected on the screen, as words or images.
7. From the front row, you are so close that you almost have to squint to see the screen clearly.
8. Imagine getting up and moving to the back row of the theater. Sit down and look at the screen again. From this far-away vantage point, notice how the nature of the thoughts and feelings projected on the screen become a little more clear as you are more removed from them.
9. Watch the thoughts and feelings on the screen for a few minutes, as if they belonged to someone else. How wondrous the human mind is, that can generate all this output!

10. Now, we are going to practice *Upeksha*, which is the Sanskrit word loosely translated as rising above or detaching.

11. Imagine you are standing outside in any setting that feels safe and pleasant.

12. Imagine you begin to rise up slowly into the sky. You feel safe.

13. Look down and see the earth, people you know, places you've been, places you would like to go.

14. Observe this quotidian reality, from this elevated place as the witness. Spend a few minutes here marveling at the beauty and complexity of the world, as if you're seeing it for the first time.

15. Finally, bring your attention back to yourself. Turn inward and imagine yourself inside your own body, sitting on a golden throne.

16. Look around and observe the different parts of your inner landscape. What does it look like in there?

17. Spend a few minutes imagining your interior landscape. Imagine emotions, memories, thoughts, plans, as material objects or clouds floating in that space. See them from a place of safety, as things that are familiar but not within you in this moment. You are the witness.

18. Take a deep breath in, exhale, and now, think about which of these methods worked best for you: witnessing the breath, seeing your thoughts and feelings on a screen, the *Upeksha* of looking down from an elevated view, or the subtle internal witness.

19. Return to any of these methods if you want to, or just stay within the space of your internal landscape, neutrally observing until the timer goes off.

20. Take another deep breath in, exhale fully, and take a moment to recognize the part of your consciousness that judges your experience. Honor that as part of being human, and also, recognize that as just one view of consciousness. Shift back to a witness perspective, and honor that experience as well.

21. Very slowly, fold your hands in front of your heart, bow your head, and make a wish or a blessing that you can take this capacity of perspective shifting and seeing value from the point of view of the witness into the real world throughout the rest of your day.

22. Lower your hands, lift your chin, and gently open your eyes. Notice any difference in how you feel.

WEEK FOUR: TWENTY MINUTES

Welcome to week four, the most advanced week. During this week, you'll expand your introversion practice to daily sessions of twenty minutes. This is actually a standard amount of time for experienced meditators, but it's hard to start at twenty minutes, which is why we've worked up to it.

The guided meditations for this week are the most advanced in this book, which might be exciting or interesting to you. If not—if these feel too "woo woo" or difficult for you—you can instead do any type of practice you've already tried so far that you enjoy, but extend the time to twenty minutes.

A reminder that this is a long time to sit still, so you can always move, stretch, stand up, or even take a break if you need to. Also remember: a wandering mind only means that you have thoughts in your head, as we all do. It's not a sign of doing anything wrong, or even of being less advanced. Even the most advanced meditators can have wandering thoughts. You will reap all the benefits of your meditation, no matter how vigorously those puppies on the playground are playing on any given day. Just keep at it because as I've said time and again, the real benefits, the big shifts, the realizations, and the wisdom come from the regular practice, not necessarily the "success" or quality of any individual practice.

One last note: You can set a timer for twenty minutes for these practices, and I've cued you to do that, but if you find that you don't have a problem staying in these practices for twenty minutes and you don't want to be interrupted with the sound of the timer going off, you can go without it. Some people really enjoy spending a longer time in these immersive experiences.

DAY ONE: *Creator of Worlds*

In this meditation, you will play the role of someone who can create entire worlds. This requires some imagination, but it's great for generating creative energy.

1. Sit or lie down comfortably, supported if necessary. Set a timer for twenty minutes.
2. Close your eyes and take a few calming breaths.
3. Now, imagine that you are a creator of worlds. You have decided to create a world today. Begin by thinking what kind of world you would like to create.
4. Imagine that simply with the power of your mind, you can manifest a world. This can be a world where you are in charge, you are the protagonist, and everything that exists in that world is something you chose to create and put there.
5. Now, imagine you begin creating the world. See it forming. Imagine shaping it you're your hands, then expanding it. What will you put on it? Imagine all the things you'll do, and imagine creating the entire environment.
6. Spend as much time as you want in this state. Let your imagination expand. Make your world as detailed as possible.
7. When you feel that your world is created to your satisfaction, slowly open your eyes.
8. Look around you and imagine that the external world you live in is also a world you personally have created. See this world as something completely of your own devising.

Imagine all its aspects are emerging right in front of you, and they were all your idea and your manifestation. Spend some time here, keeping your eyes open or closing them again, imagining how the external world looks and feels different when you see it as your own creation.

9. Now, close your eyes again if you haven't already, and using the inspiration from the external world, continue to create the inner world you were working on before. Approach this with a sense of playful whimsy. What will you add? What will you change? Will it spin in space next to our planet, or somewhere far away? What kind of influence will you have? What are its physical laws, the nature of its inhabitants? Stay here for as long as you like.

10. If you still have time, open your eyes again and playfully experience the outer world you imagine you have created, imagining how you might alter things based on inspiration from the world you were just creating. Continue to go back and forth between these two worlds a few more times, feeling ownership over and joyfully reveling in the worlds you have created, until the timer goes off.

11. Take a deep breath and bring your hands together in front of your heart in a prayer position. Bow your head and honor your creative abilities. Consider how true it really is that you create your own world. Honor that discovery, or rediscovery.

12. Slowly lower your hands and open your eyes. Notice in what ways the world looks different, in the moment and for the rest of the day.

DAY TWO: *Advanced Relaxation Meditation*

Sometimes, getting your entire body and mind to relax can feel like the most difficult thing in the world. If you feel some frustration, know that you are planting the seeds of relaxation for later. This can be a process. Or, you may find it easy to do. Everyone has a different experience. For me, one of the most important parts of introversions is to create an environment of safety and welcoming. You'll be creating that space in this practice.

1. Sit or lie down comfortably, supported as necessary. Set a timer for twenty minutes.

2. Close your eyes and begin to slow and deepen your breathing. Take a few minutes to feel the effect of slower, deeper breaths.

3. Imagine the room is filled with people (and/or animals) you love and feel safe around. You are all meditating together. Imagine opening your heart and generously welcoming all you have chosen to imagine in the room with you, and feel the warmth as they welcome you as well.

4. Consider that relaxation is a journey and you can embark upon this journey with hope and patience. First you will prepare your body to move towards a relaxed state.

5. Begin by visualizing your pelvis as a bowl. Breathing in through your nose, imagine the breath as a sweet nectar that flows down and pools in the bowl of the pelvis. Feel this for a few minutes.

6. With each breath in, continue to fill the pelvis with this sweet nectar. Imagine your pelvis begins to feel heavy and anchored with the weight of the nectar.

7. Now, imagine that your spine is like a tree rising up from the bowl of the pelvis. Visualize your spine as a strong, fortified core rising through your torso and through the crown of your head. Stay here feeling the strength and fortitude of the nectar-filled bowl and the trunk of your spine.

8. Next, imagine a beautiful valley surrounded by mountains, covered in lush grasses and wildflowers.

9. Now, imagine that in the middle of this field is a simple, sturdy table. On top of the table, visualize a crystal ball. Approach the table and look into the crystal ball.

10. In the crystal ball, you see something about your reality— a relationship, a goal, a stress, a memory, an experience, a success. Or, it might move through different scenes in your life.

11. A beautiful throne appears in front of the table. This throne is magical and can float. Sit down on the throne and feel the throne beginning to rise above and a little away from the table and the crystal ball.

12. Look down from above and see the crystal ball, still showing reality, but from afar. The images begin to have less power over you as you rise above them. You feel completely safe and you have complete control over the throne as you rise a little higher up and a little farther away.

13. Look back again, down to the almost imperceptible crystal ball. It's still there, but it has very little effect on you anymore.

14. Now, bring all your attention to the experience of sitting in this magical throne, floating above the mountains and

the valley, bathing in the light of the sun. You feel softer, having let go of your daily reality. Just exist here, in this soft safe light, until the timer goes off.

15. Take a deep breath in, then a slow full exhale as you imagine the throne coming back down and fading away. Feel yourself back in the room where you are.

16. Bring your palms together in front of your heart and bow your head. Give yourself a moment of recognition that you planted seeds for relaxation, now or in the future.

17. Release your hands down and gently open your eyes. Notice any change in how relaxed your body feels.

DAY THREE: The Marble Exercise

This is a more advanced variation on the body scan introversion. I call this a directional attention introversion. Instead of working your way through the body as you relax it, you'll be focusing on moving an imaginary marble around to different parts of your body, and focusing on that. Although people who love visualization can easily imagine the marble, this introversion is more about feeling, not seeing, and you don't have to know what the inside of your body looks like to try this.

1. Sit comfortably, supported if necessary. Set a timer for twenty minutes.

2. Close your eyes and take a few calming breaths.

3. Now, slowly and easily, think about your left index finger. Bring your attention to this finger. Move it slightly if you need help really zeroing in on it.

4. Once you've got the feeling of it (keep your eyes closed), try to picture the space inside your left index finger, at the tip, and imagine there is a small marble in that space. Spend some time feeling the marble inside the tip of your finger.

5. When you've got it, imagine the marble dissolves, and then reconfigures behind your right eyeball. Focus on that small spot in that one very specific area. See if you can feel it, or at least get a sense of it.

6. Once you've got the feeling of the marble behind your eye, imagine it dissolves again, then reconfigures in the center of your stomach. See if you can imagine moving it around slightly. Even if you can't physically feel it, just try to get the sense of it, as well as you can.

7. The marble dissolves again, then reappears inside your left big toe. Let it stay there for a while until you sense it.

8. Now you get to choose. Put the marble somewhere really obscure: the bottom of the butt cheek on the right side, the far left edge of your left collar bone, between your bottom two ribs, your choice.

9. Each time you get a good sense of where the marble is, move it around again, to other very specific parts of your body. You can imagine it dissolves and reappears, or you can feel it moving slowly, gently through your body from place to place.

10. After you've done this for a while, let the marble slowly dissolve away. Keep doing this until the timer goes off.

11. Take a deep breath, slowly open your eyes, and reorient yourself. Consider whether you feel any different after doing this exercise.

DAY FOUR: Emotional Focus Meditation

In this meditation, you'll be looking at some of the more difficult parts of your consciousness so you can practice moving through them. This practice can help these emotions to feel more accessible and less cloaked. In this introversion in particular, it can be more effective to sit with a straight back, regally and with sovereignty and honor, if that position is available to you. The traditional thinking is that this position conducts energy better during meditation than when your spine is not in a vertical position.

1. Sit or lie down comfortably, supported if necessary. Set a timer for twenty minutes.
2. Close your eyes and take a few deep breaths.
3. Look within, with compassion, at how you feel right now. Are you feeling calm, agitated, happy, cynical, whimsical? Whatever part of your personality feels dominant right now, recognize that as exactly right for this moment.
4. Now, imbue the seat that you are in and the air around you with an imaginary cocoon of unconditional love. You can do no wrong in this space. You are surrounded with compassion and love, no matter what your mind might be saying. This is a catalyst to a deeper meditation practice.
5. For a few moments, feel this loving space. Try to sense the *bhava*, the essential energy underneath the emotions you feel as you hold silence for yourself in this space. There is a spectrum, from the deep essential *bhava* of an emotion

to its manifested side, where you may laugh or cry or yell. Feel that spectrum that exists for every emotion.

6. Now, contemplate any shadow feelings under the surface. Are you feeling doubt, shame, guilt, regret, or anger? Feel it in your skin. Give it space. Recognize it as part of your human consciousness. Search for the *bhava* of whatever rises, as you are able. You don't have to define it. Just feel its source deep within yourself. Stay here for as long as you like, just feeling the source of those negative energies and honoring them as human.

7. Next, imagine you are breathing in forgiveness. See it as light. As you inhale, imagine every cell in your body begins to glow with this light of forgiveness. With each inhalation, offer yourself a profound forgiveness, or offer forgiveness to someone else, or say to yourself: *I hold the capacity to forgive, when I am ready, when it's appropriate.*

8. Feel the deep essential *bhava* of forgiveness glowing inside of you. Stay here for as long as you like.

9. Now, feel a flower at the base of your spine, growing and rising up through your body as it blooms and keeps blooming, with layers and layers of blossoms. This is a flower of gratitude, rising within you. You don't have to accept it or interact with it. Just feel it as available to you always, rising out of the *bhava* of gratitude.

10. Take a deep cleansing breath in, then release it making the sound *haaaa*. Take another deep cleansing breath, releasing it again with the sound *haaaa*.

11. Fold your hands in front of your heart. Bow your head. Bring this awareness of the sources of unconditional

love, forgiveness, and gratitude with you into the rest of
your day.

12. Lower your hands, raise your head, and open your eyes.
    Notice any difference in how you feel.

DAY FIVE: Ekagrata Meditation

There are a lot of incredible practices that feel like bending an illusion
towards reality. This is one of them. In this advanced introversion,
you will focus on a particular thing and play with the idea that you
aren't actually seeing that thing, but only seeing an image in your
mind of that thing. If this is true, then you can move that image
wherever you choose. You will envision the brain as a reflective screen
projecting the image behind your eyes.

Don't worry if you can't achieve all aspects of this introversion.
This isn't about doing it "right." It's about throwing open the doors
of your focus and perception to reveal the potential of the mind.
Many people believe they are good at focusing until they try this
meditation! When you can keep your attention intensely focused,
you can eventually feel that you have merged with that object of
your concentration. By the end of this inspirational meditation,
deep focus will become an exciting and rewarding goal. I find this
one quite challenging, but I won't assume it will be challenging
for you.

1. Sit comfortably, with support if needed. Set a timer for
   twenty minutes.
2. Take a few deep, slow breaths.
3. Begin by holding your arm out straight in front of you,
   fingers pointed up. Look at one of your fingertips.

4. Close your eyes and see the image of your fingertip in your mind. Consider that the image is not actually there. Your mind is creating it. You're not actually seeing your fingertip outside of yourself. You're seeing it inside of yourself.

5. Now open your eyes. Look at your fingertip again. Still, you are seeing the finger inside of yourself, as a projected image in your eye. This image is just light that has to travel to you for you to see it. Think about how the light is traveling to your eye.

6. Now, look at a space about halfway between your fingertip and your eye. Imagine the light traveling through that space. What if you could stop the light in the middle?

7. Now, try to place that image of your fingertip that exists in your mind, into the middle of the space between your actual fingertip and your eye.

8. Now, look at the space halfway between the middle space where you have placed the image of your fingertip, dividing the space between the image and your eye in half again. Try to place that image in that space.

9. When you've got it, divide the space in half again, and put the image there.

10. Continue dividing the space again and again. How far (or how close) can you go?

11. Contemplate as you do this that no matter how many times you divide the space, the image will never actually get all the way to your eye.

12. You can now begin to double the space, until the image of your fingertip reaches its original placement. Go back

and forth, doubling and halving, as you move the image between your fingertip and your eye at will. Continue to do this, maintaining your focus, or redirecting it back if your mind wanders, until the timer goes off.

13. Take a deep breath and slowly open your eyes. As you look around the space where you are, consider that everything you see is merely an image projected via light to the back of your eye...so how fixed can any of it really be? Let yourself wonder about this.

14. Notice if reality looks different now. Take this wonderment with you throughout the rest of your day.

DAY SIX: Advanced Breathwork

In yoga, the practice of *Pranayama* can get quite advanced, but this exercise is just a little more complex than some of the other breathwork practices in this book.

While I always advocate breathing in whatever way feels comfortable and doesn't make you feel anxious, there is nose breathing... This exercise is best practiced while sitting with an upright spine, as well as you are able.

1. Sit comfortably, supported naturally. Set a timer for twenty minutes.

2. Begin by breathing naturally. This is more challenging than it sounds. It can be difficult not to control your breath once you start noticing it. However, there is a depth and pace of the breath that is almost programmed into you at any given moment. See if you can follow your breath, rather than leading it. Stay here for a few

moments, simply tuning in as intensely as you can on what your breath is doing, but standing back metaphorically to observe rather than control. If you feel like you need to breathe in and out of your nose or mouth or both, that's fine. Do whatever your body wants to do naturally.

3. Place your right hand on your chest and exert a slight pressure so that as you breathe into your chest, you feel the breath lifting your hand with your inhalation, and lowering your hand with your exhalation. Try to imagine your hand is buoyant, floating up and down as if on water, up with the inhale, down with the exhale.

4. As you inhale, try to maintain the expansion in your breath, even when you exhale. Imagine your chest continues to expand with each breath.

5. Switch hands and feel your left hand floating buoyantly on the breath. Stay here as long as feels good, continuing to feel that expansion in your chest.

6. Now, lower your hands and put your hands right at the base of your ribs with your thumb pointing back and your fingers pointing forward. Try breathing into the area where your hands are, allowing the rib cage to gently expand and contract, opening on the inhale, closing on the exhale.

7. As with your chest, try to feel the ribs continuing to expand, even with the exhale. Stay here for a few minutes.

8. Now, reach your hands back, placing your thumbs on your low back around where your kidneys are, with your fingers to the front. Breath into the lowest part of your lungs, even feeling your diaphragm expanding and contracting with each breath.

9. Again, try to feel the expansion, even as you exhale. Stay here for a few minutes.

10. Release your hands to your thighs and breathe naturally again for a moment or two.

11. Now, maintaining a sense of expansion in your mind, take a very deep inhale.

12. Hold the breath and feel a light, expansive floating feeling as you hold for about five seconds.

13. Gently and deeply exhale.

14. Inhale again, trying to breathe in an even deeper breath. Hold the breath, again for about five seconds, feeling an expansive floating. Exhale gently and deeply.

15. One more time, inhale, expand, and hold. Exhale fully.

16. Ease back into your natural breath.

17. Continue to sit, feeling the effect of this breathwork throughout your body, until the timer goes off.

18. Fold your palms together in front of your heart and bow your head. Offer gratitude for this practice and for the energy and calm that the breath can bring into your body.

19. Lower your hands, raise your head, and gently open your eyes. Notice any difference in how you feel.

DAY SEVEN: Connection Consciousness

For the last practice in week four, I'd like to bring your focus back to the connection that is such a valuable benefit of introversion. Cultivating a sense of connection and empathy is something I like to approach with humility and respect. Empathy in particular is a connector. It helps us to see things from a wider perspective, beyond our natural and justifiable self-interest. We all have this and should never feel guilty about it, but self-interest can become so cloistered that we lose our awareness of the experiences other people are having. When we lose this, our own self-interest, almost paradoxically, becomes limited. Conversely, by stretching our antennae to consider that someone else might be having the same dreams, hopes, and fears as we do—and not just to feel it sympathetically but to actually feel it empathetically—we gain a kind of satiating, peaceful, weighty, safe oasis within. There is some kind of reaction we get when we connect through empathy, then turn back inside—we feel a little more okay. And that is the gateway to elevated living.

1. Sit or lie down comfortably, supported if necessary. Set a timer for twenty minutes.
2. Close your eyes and begin to listen to the natural movement of the breath. Stay here for a few minutes, and gradually slow and deepen your breath.
3. Imagine all the people in the world who might be introverting in any way at this moment, looking within to find wisdom or peace. Feel the shared energy, like a web across the planet, with glowing lights wherever someone is turning inward.
4. Imagine sending a deep, sincere longing for love, support, and connection throughout this network, touching each person and spreading across the network of shared energy. Stay here for a few minutes, feeling the natural waves of light moving over the world.

5. Now, putting your skeptical mind to the side for a moment, open yourself up to the possibility that you can sense the energy of how each person in this network feels. You can scan across the web of lights, stopping on any light and feeling the emotions of that person. Spend some time scanning the web of introversion, stopping here and there at different lights and connecting with that person energetically.

6. Next, imagine pausing at one of the lights, someone you don't know and have never met, and sending out a signal: *Who are you? How are you?*

7. Feel for the answer. Notice what comes across.

8. Imagine that person sending the signal back: *Who are you? How are you?* Send your answer energetically outward towards that person.

9. Spend more time exploring this web of light, sending, receiving, and honoring all who seek connection. Feel that energetic connection moving from you to every other person and back to you. You are all connected by energy and light. Stay here until the timer goes off.

10. Take a deep breath and slowly let the image fade, but see if you can feel the energetic connection to all humanity, through which we are all light, and all come from the same light.

11. Fold your hands in front of your heart and bow your head in reverence to this light that is always there and always within every living thing, even when we don't see or feel it.

12. Slowly lower your hands, raise your head, and open your eyes.

13. Make a wish that you can carry this sense of connection with you throughout your day, your week, even your whole life, and that some part of you never forgets that no matter what differences you encounter in others, the same light glows deep inside us all.

CHAPTER 10

MORE TURNING-IN PRACTICES

In this chapter I've set out a number of different introversions, or turning-in practices, that you can pick and choose from, depending on what resonates with you and which ones have the most utility. I recommend reviewing the chapter on how to prepare for meditation a few times, so you really set yourself up for success. Do your best to remember that introversion and meditation really can be a lifelong practice, helping you to step out of your normal urgency, agenda-oriented mindset and see your meditation as part of a long process of growth and unveiling of your inner self. That especially goes for days when you have a bad meditation day (not unlike a bad hair day). Do your best to see even the days when you struggle in your practice as planting seeds that will bear fruit later, and ultimately, remind yourself there's no way to meditate incorrectly.

RELAXATION INTROVERSION

This introversion is great to do as part of a warm-down after vigorous exercise, or for when you're feeling stressed. It's also a nice way to wind down at the end of a busy day. This relaxation starts in a sitting position, then ends lying down, so it can help you ease into sleep. You can also do this exercise in bed at night.

1. Begin by sitting comfortably with your back against a wall or supported by bolsters, cushions, pillows, blankets, or whatever you need.

2. Close your eyes and take a few deep, nourishing breaths. Think about drawing your attention inward, drinking in the inhale along with your focus. Remember, there is no way you can do this wrong. Stay here for a few minutes, just breathing and nourishing yourself with the sacred nectar that is the breath.

3. Without trying to slow down your thoughts, step apart from them and begin to watch them, as if they are puppies wrestling or children playing on a playground. Watch them for a few minutes.

4. Imagine yourself sitting on a park bench watching, on a perfect sunny day at the perfect temperature. Just breathe, watch your thoughts with benevolent interest, and pretend you can feel the warmth of the sun on your skin. Bathe in the light. Stay here for a few minutes.

5. Slowly, if you desire, shift your position so you are lying down comfortably and supported. Or, you can stay seated if you like.

6. Bring your attention to the crown of your head, and let your scalp and forehead relax. Feel a relaxation in your temples and into your ears. Feel your eyes heavy in their sockets, sinking down into a relaxed state.

7. Soften your jaw, releasing all clenching. Let your tongue relax. Feel it sinking down.

8. Move your attention to your collarbones and chest. Relax your shoulders and chest muscles. Feel the warm relaxation spreading down the arms, into the elbows, and into the hands. Let your hands relax and sink, as if they were each holding a heavy, precious jewel.

9. Let go of all tension in your belly and in the sides of the hips. Stay here as long as you like. Whenever you feel tension creeping back in anywhere, bring your attention to that spot and release, letting the tension fade away.

10. Soften your knees and let go of all tension in your calf muscles, ankles, and feet. Let your feet relax as if you are bathing them in warm water.

11. Let the weight of your entire body sink gently into the floor, heavy, calm, at peace. Give yourself permission to relax completely.

12. Stay here and let your mind sink into sleep. Or, slowly bend your knees and roll to the side, then slowly sit up. Take a deep breath in, exhale slowly, and notice the ways your body and mind feel different. Are you calmer, more relaxed, more focused? Recognize that this ease and calm ultimately comes from within.

13. Gently open your eyes.

THAT BEING SAID . . .

While there is no way to do introversion wrong, it can feel frustrating. You can have trouble regulating the breath or feeling calm or sitting still. As you begin to introvert more regularly, see if you can bring your awareness to when introversion feels easier and when it feels more challenging.

Your difficulty may have to do with how much sleep you got, what happened to you that day, or whether you are simply feeling in a more heightened nervous system state. On those days when it feels more difficult, I encourage you to sink into a feeling of patience and forgiveness for yourself. See if you can pull back and see your churning thoughts with a sense of wonder. What a brain you have, to be able to think with such complexity and speed!

When you step apart and become radically accepting of, and even impressed by your thoughts, you may feel your entire body relaxing and your nervous system slowing down. Or not! Either way, bring awareness to it and try to see it neutrally, as a benevolent observer.

INTROVERSION FOR PATIENCE

This introversion is actually pretty tough for me personally. I struggle with patience, which is why I like to do this meditation and offer it for those of us who struggle with this state of mind. This introversion seeks to balance what we experience on the outside with what we feel on the inside. Rather than superimposing an "I should be patient" kind of mentality, the purpose of this introversion is to stop vilifying impatience and accept that it's part of the human experience. I don't condone impatience—I think we can all agree that it's useful to cultivate patience. But I also want to honor that impatience is common to the human experience.

1. Sit comfortably, supported as necessary. If you feel a lack of patience with sitting still (ha!), don't try to force an uncomfortable or strenuous position. Also, although I recommend doing this meditation with closed eyes, open them if you feel you need to open them.

2. Let your deep, slow breath invite you inward. Stay here for a few minutes, just feeling the breath opening a doorway into your internal landscape.

3. Feel the air around you in the room. Imagine that within the air around you is the energy of urgency, as well as enthusiasm. Recognize if you feel discomfort around the feeling of urgency. Let the impatience exist around you, as if it's something you could breathe in, if you chose.

4. Notice that with the impatience also exists an energy of calm wisdom.

5. Using your breath, turn in towards the center of your chest around your heart. Breathe this calm wisdom into the space around your heart. Feel that the impatient energy is still there, but it is outside of you, not within you. You can choose not to take it in.

6. Feel the inner patience filling your heart. Stay here for as long as you like, letting the patience infuse your body with a calm sense of timelessness.

7. Take a deep breath in, then exhale fully.

8. Spend a moment in recognition of your experience in this introversion. Acknowledge that no matter what your exact experience of this meditation was, you have planted the seeds of patience in your heart.

9. Fold your hands in front of your heart, bow your head, and make a wish: that the seeds of patience can also flow forward into someone else who needs them.

10. Release your hands and gently open your eyes.

INTROVERSION FOR COURAGE

In this introversion, I don't want to superimpose the idea or mentality of courage onto you. Instead, I'd like you to think about the aspect of courage that is resilience. Trusting in our capacity to face our fears with resilience creates an inner brand of courage that can carry you through your next challenge.

1. Sit comfortably with support if necessary. Sit up tall and close your eyes.

2. Deepen and slow your breathing. Listen to your breath moving in and out of your body.

3. With a childlike sense of fun, allow your thoughts to dance through your mind without judgment. Feel compassion for your many thoughts, as if you are watching them play. Stay here for a few minutes.

4. Begin to contemplate the idea that your capacity to be resilient is a kind of courage. It's human to be afraid to face your fears because you think you might not be able

to handle them, but see if you can feel an inner resilience, or that feeling that you are internally strong and can endure challenges.

5. Feel compassion for your own fears and doubts. There is nothing wrong with fear or doubt. You don't need to push these feelings away. They are natural responses.

6. Imagine your spinal column as a source of resilience, or inner strength.

7. Imagine a tree with roots in your pelvis, growing down into the earth.

8. Imagine the trunk rising up through your core and through the crown of your head, where its branches expand upward.

9. Imagine this tree contains a column of light that extends down into the earth, up through your core, and out the crown of your head.

10. Soften your face and feel that inner strength in your core. This is resilience. Feel this in whatever way it's happening for you. Stay here for a few minutes, taking in this inner core of strength.

11. Feel the resilience expanding out in all directions, lighting up the rest of your body. Bask in this feeling of strength and light for a few minutes.

12. Take a deep breath in, then exhale fully. Sit in silence as the visual of the tree and the beam of light fade away. Notice if you feel stronger, more resilient, or more courageous.

13. Fold your hands in front of your heart and bow your head. Feel gratitude for this practice.

14. Release your hands down and gently open your eyes.

INTROVERSION FOR EMPATHY

Empathy is complicated. It sounds simple—to relate to or share the emotions of someone else. But that's easier said than done and has many versions and facets. I don't want to impose my ideas of empathy onto you. I hope you will use this introversion to discover what empathy means for you. I would like you to think about how radical acceptance is tied with empathy, and that a "should" mentality is tied with a lack of empathy. I would argue that empathy isn't always the right choice. That being said, the skilled cultivation of empathy is the purpose of this introversion.

1. Find a comfortable position, supported if necessary. Close your eyes.
2. Breathe for a few moments and feel your breath moving in and out of you, without judgment or control.
3. Think of someone you've had trouble understanding, or who you feel needs your empathy. Or, consider whether you would like to generate more empathy towards a particular group, or humans in general.
4. Imagine a series of words coming into your mind, like slides in a slide show. Contemplate each word and whether it feels like empathy to you:
   - Compassion
   - Patience
   - Sensitivity
   - Acceptance
   - Forgiveness
   - Love

5. Think about which of these words resonated with you, or seemed to light up as you viewed it. Consider how that word might be a bridge to manifesting empathy within you.

6. Feel that word. Can it generate an internal sense of empathy for someone in particular, or for people in general? Sit here for a few minutes, contemplating these words.

7. Take a deep breath in, then exhale fully.

8. Consider whether anything within you feels changed or transformed. Does empathy feel more accessible to you than it did before, or have you simply planted the seeds of empathy, laying the groundwork for a more foundational sense of empathy in your life?

9. Fold your hands in front of your heart, bow your head, and send your empathy unconditionally, as well as you can, outward.

10. Release your hands and gently open your eyes.

INTROVERSION FOR HEALING

I'd love for you to approach this meditation with the recognition that healing can mean many things and will mean different things to different people. However my words may sound to you, I ask that you think of healing in whatever capacity you need right now. Anxiety, agita, stress, pain, suffering, trauma—these are broad manifestations of negative energies that exist. Recognizing these exist empowers us to face them rather than fear them. One of the ways to do that is to just breathe.

1. Sit comfortably, supported if necessary, and close your eyes.

2. Breathe naturally, in and out, quietly listening to your breath and feeling it moving in and out. Let your breath gently draw your attention inward.

3. Slow your breath down a bit, to help you feel more grounded in this moment.

4. Soften the muscles of your face.

5. Soften the muscles of your upper back.

6. Even as you sit tall, see if you can feel a buoyancy and openness in your upper body, throughout chest and shoulders.

7. Feel a mysterious and humble spaciousness within your body, with the recognition that the feeling of health is, in a way, mysterious. Stay here for a few minutes.

8. If you are presently in a state of pain or if you are going through something and the idea of healing feels a little scary, feel your spine as rigid and stable, as if you have an inner core of profound fortitude.

9. At the same time, allow the outer boundaries of your body—your skin and muscles—to be soft and to feel almost fluid.

10. Feel this openness on the outside and the fortitude on the inside.

11. Now, imagine the room you are in has golden, lustrous walls. The room has such beauty and depth that it feels warm and rich. For a few minutes, sit and absorb the light of this room, which is imbued with healing, loving energy. Imagine this absorption is healing. Stay here for a few minutes, letting in that golden light.

12. Now, begin to turn the light of the room into a bright white light.

13. Imagine the light glowing, closer and closer to you, then moving inside of you, where the light coalesces into a brilliant blue pearl in the center of your heart. Luminous, resplendent, potent. Absorb this healing light from the blue pearl for as long as you need, feeling that healing pulsating from the inside out.

14. Take a deep breath in through your nose, then exhale through your mouth. Do this three times.

15. Fold your hands in front of your heart, bow your head, and take a moment to ask for, be thankful for, or recognize any healing you feel. Or maybe you feel a simple expansion of your capacity to heal.

16. Send that healing energy out to someone who needs healing.

17. Release your hands, and open your eyes.

INTROVERSION FOR A BETTER NIGHT'S SLEEP

I do many sleep meditations on the Peloton app because they are the most requested and most popular. Falling and staying asleep is indeed a challenge for many people. My hope is that this meditation can become habitual for you and make your sleep feel deeper, more healing, more rejuvenating, and sweeter. Since this is a sleep meditation, I recommend either recording this meditation or reading it over enough times that you get the gist of it and can do it on your own, in bed, with your eyes closed.

Before you begin, get everything ready for sleep. That may mean turning off any devices, putting on whatever you want to wear to bed, and basically taking care of everything you would normally take care of, just in case you fall asleep during the meditation. You can do this meditation sitting on the floor with your back against the wall, or in bed with your back against wall or headboard. Or, you can do it lying down. In this meditation, I'll use a number of different techniques to slow down and settle the body and mind, easing them into rest. Instead of forcing calm, these techniques will allow calm to permeate and settle naturally.

1. Begin by noticing your breath. As you inhale, say to yourself, "This is my inhale." As you exhale, say to yourself, "This is my exhale." Do this for a few minutes.

2. Now, imagine the room you're in, even the neighborhood you're in—the entire physical space around you—as warm and safe.

3. Translate that feeling of safety and warmth inside, as you turn inward towards your internal landscape. See it and feel it as safe and warm.

4. Deepen your breath, lengthening your inhalation and exhalation.

5. Notice the thoughts passing through your mind, seemingly arising from nowhere. Imagine that your thoughts are voices. In the same way you would listen to a song, listen to your thoughts.

6. Now, list the thoughts as you notice them. If you are thinking about your to-do list, make an actual list in your mind. If you are thinking about things you did today or sometime in the past, make a list of those things. Let your thoughts settle through the simple process of organization.

7. Now, label the thoughts in categories. Allow a thought to arise, then decide what kind of thought it is: an emotion, a memory, a regret, a hope, a task. Whatever it is, simply label it and allow the next thought to arise.

8. Take a deep breath in, and exhale fully. Notice if you feel any shift in how your body or mind feels.

9. Now, imagine your body is becoming heavier. Feel the weight of impending sleep gently settling into you.

10. Imagine a warm waterfall above you, gently flowing over your body, washing away all the experiences of the day with its cleansing, nourishing water. The water flows from the top of your head, over your shoulders, down your back, over your hips, down your legs, all the way down to your feet, and all the experiences of the day flow down and away.

11. Feel this cleansing from your crown to your feet as the warm water continues to flow over you, washing you clean. Feel the water flowing over you for as long as you want to stay there.

12. Now, begin to feel a soft, melting sensation, from head to shoulders to back to hips to legs to feet. Let yourself feel this warm, melting sensation flowing through you for as long as you need.

13. If you're still awake, and you aren't in bed yet, very slowly ease yourself into bed and drift off to sleep.

14. Sweet dreams!

I'll close out this chapter by saying that ultimately, meditation is about what you find inside of you, not about what I tell you. It doesn't matter whether I tell you it will work for you or not. It is soul work for you and you alone, but it can be a beautiful way to build a bridge between your daily life and a deeper experience. It is the inner wisdom that's doing the teaching. All I'm proposing here is that you entertain the idea that it's a little bit easier than you think, that it can become a little more prominent in your life than you think, that you can become more present than you think, and that this practice of introverting will become even more profound than you think.

A BLESSING

As we come to the end of this book, I want to say clearly that I can't claim anything I've passed along will be one 100 percent true for you. For me, it feels very close to the truth because of the wisdom of my teachers, my own contemplation, and ultimately, the harmonic resonance that it has to me. This gets me pretty close to saying that what I say in this book is true. The essence of introversion is for your truth to be revealed to you from within.

I'd also like to leave you with a blessing. One of the things I loved most about going to church was the preacher's blessing or benediction at the end of the service. Even as a kid, it resonated with me as kind and benevolent.

The words of this blessing are reminders of your greatness. I understand if, when you read it or say it to yourself, you might doubt whether it's true for you. The words might not resonate with you, and that's okay. But I can say with all my heart that even if these are not the right words for you, I believe in your goodness and your greatness. I believe in your humanity and your divinity. I believe in your sovereignty and your freedom.

Therefore, my parting blessing to you is:

> *May you always remember your true self as an infinite source of love and grace.*
> *May you always remember that it is your birthright to live your truth.*
> *May you always remember that the vicissitudes of the world can never extinguish your inner peace.*
> *And may you always remember that you are filled with the fortitude and the power to continually become more of who you already are.*

ACKNOWLEDGMENTS

Writing this book has been one of the absolute joys of my life, and also one of the most difficult things I've ever done. It could never have happened without the support and influence of many—and that begins with my mom, Jan Runkel, who taught me many of my greatest lessons and is always there for me.

I don't know what I would do without the support of friends, who constantly hold me up, keep me positive, and are the scaffolding for my optimism and enduring sense of hope. Many of these are yoga colleagues who are friends as well, especially Mindy Bacharach, Tiffany Fraser, Marc Holzman, Andrea Boni, Tara Judelle, Elena Brower, Seane Corn, Maryl Baldridge, and my dear friends Hunter Jackson, Wilson Cruz, Wesley Adams, Todd Sears, Chun Rosencranz, Paul McGill, and Robbie Fairchild.

My teachers and other professional yoga and meditation colleagues have made an indelible impression on me and helped me to form and express the underlying philosophies in this book. Those include my mentor Sally Kempton, who recently passed on from this life and whose presence I both grieve and still perceive. Also, in the yoga sphere, John Friend, Desiree Rumbaugh, Sara Ivanhoe, Sue Elkind, Naime Jezzeny, Anthony Benenati, Bryan Kest, Maty Ezraty, Lisa Wolford, and Michelle Marchildon. And my other meditation teachers Paul Muller-Ortega, Carlos Pomeda, Douglas Brooks, and Christopher "Hareesh" Wallis.

Thanks are also due to my amazing publishing team. Thanks to my agent, Alex Glass, for believing in me and moving this book from the idea I had in my head to the pages of this actual physical book. Thanks to my editor, Renée Sedliar, who has been so deeply kind, supportive, and involved in not just the text but the innermost spirit of what this book is and what it seeks to achieve. Also, thanks to the wonderful Amanda Kain, whose creativity and support have meant the world, as well as Kara Brammer, Lauren Rosenthal, Mary Ann Naples, Nzinga Temu, Fred Francis, and Bart Dawson. Many thanks to my social media manager, Sean Azari, for making my analog heart visible in a digital world. And this book never would have happened without Eve Adamson, my cowriter—thanks to her for her wit, skill, discipline, and for our incredible joyful synchronicity, which always surprises us both.

I probably wouldn't even be in a position to write a book if not for the platform Peloton has afforded me. All my fellow instructors, especially Tunde Oyeneyin, Ally Love, Robin Arzon, Ben Alldis, Cody Rigsby, Emma Lovewell, and Alex Toussaint. My yoga and meditation colleagues: Kristin McGee, Anna Greenberg, Aditi Shah, Denis Morton, Dr. Chelsea Jackson Roberts, Mariana Fernandez, Kirra Michel, and Nico Sarani. To the senior leadership at Peloton, particularly Jen Cotter, Amanda Hill, Britton Schey, and to the entire Peloton family on both sides of the screen.

Finally, last and most of all, my deepest gratitude and my whole heart go out to my husband Chris—my rock and the love of my life.

INDEX

ABOUT ROSS RAYBURN

Ross Rayburn first discovered yoga after experiencing a sports-related knee injury over twenty years ago. At the time, he was barely flexible enough to touch his toes! He soon discovered the healing and transformative properties of yoga and decided to commit to the practice fully.

Ross became a scholar of physical healing, diving deep into biomechanics and the inner workings of the human body. He first trained in Ashtanga and Iyengar Yoga in 1999 and became a certified Anusara Yoga teacher in 2003. In 2004, he opened YogaInsideOut in Los Angeles and in 2007, he went on the road full-time, teaching workshops and trainings all around the world. Ross has traveled to more than thirty countries to teach, and loves connecting people with diverse backgrounds through yoga.

He began teaching yoga and meditation for Peloton in 2018, and today he is the Lead Instructor of Yoga and Meditation for Peloton. In his classes, Ross invites his students to tap into their authentic selves through movement, exploring the strength of the human spirit along the way. He is known for teaching some of the most sophisticated aspects of yoga with passion, humor, and clarity and is renowned for his knowledge and skill in helping people with physical injuries.

Ross has worked with a number of professional athletes and dancers, and internationally he has taught meditation and therapeutic trainings to hundreds of teachers and students including physical therapists and medical doctors.

Ross lives in New York City with his husband, the director/choreographer Christopher Wheeldon. Connect with Ross on Instagram (@RossRayburnYoga), or get to know more about him and check his class schedule at https://www.onepeloton.com/instructors/yoga.